Get Healthy
SINGAPORE
IT'S TIME TO WAKE UP!

Vismai Schonfelder
Chiropractor

TUTTLE Publishing

Tokyo | Rutland, Vermont | Singapore

The Tuttle Story
"Books to Span the East and West"

Our core mission at Tuttle Publishing is to create books which bring people together one page at a time. Tuttle was founded in 1832 in the small New England town of Rutland, Vermont (USA). Our fundamental values remain as strong today as they were then—to publish best-in-class books informing the English-speaking world about the countries and peoples of Asia. The world has become a smaller place today and Asia's economic, cultural and political influence has expanded, yet the need for meaningful dialogue and information about this diverse region has never been greater. Since 1948, Tuttle has been a leader in publishing books on the cultures, arts, cuisines, languages and literatures of Asia. Our authors and photographers have won numerous awards and Tuttle has published thousands of books on subjects ranging from martial arts to paper crafts. We welcome you to explore the wealth of information available on Asia at **www.tuttlepublishing.com**.

Published by Tuttle Publishing, an imprint of Periplus Editions (HK) Ltd

www.tuttlepublishing.com

Copyright © Vismai Schonfelder

Photograph page 68 by giedre vaitekune/ Shutterstock.
Illustration of confused man page 30 by one line man/Shutterstock. Background lettering by Heleen Dankbaar.
All other illustrations by Heleen Dankbaar.

ISBN 978 0 8048 5272 2

Printed in Malaysia   1912VP

23 22 21 20 19   10 9 8 7 6 5 4 3 2 1

Distributed by

North America, Latin America & Europe
Tuttle Publishing
364 Innovation Drive
North Clarendon, VT 05759-9436 U.S.A.
Tel: (802) 773-8930; Fax: (802) 773-6993
info@tuttlepublishing.com
www.tuttlepublishing.com

Japan
Tuttle Publishing
Yaekari Building, 3rd Floor
5-4-12 Osaki, Shinagawa-ku, Tokyo 141 0032
Tel: (81) 3 5437-0171; Fax: (81) 3 5437-0755
sales@tuttle.co.jp; www.tuttle.co.jp

Asia Pacific
Berkeley Books Pte. Ltd.
3 Kallang Sector
#04-01, Singapore 349278
Tel: (65) 6741-2178; Fax: (65) 6741-2179
inquiries@periplus.com.sg
www.tuttlepublishing.com

TUTTLE PUBLISHING* is a registered trademark of Tuttle Publishing, a division of Periplus Editions (HK) Ltd.

I dedicate my book to the humble cleverness of your body.

Today your body:
Had approximately 100,000 thoughts.
Breathed 18,720 times.
Produced about 1.5 litres of urine to clean itself of toxins.
Changed the food you ate into fuel.
Pumped 40,000 litres of water in and out of its cells.
Held its blood sugar levels to accurate levels.
Held its temperature to 37.2 degrees Celsius.
Made your heart beat 105,000 times.
Distinguished more than 1 million colour surfaces.
Inhaled more than 2 million litres of air.
Blinked 15,000 times.
Shed over 100,000 particles of skin.
Allowed your blood to travel more than 80,000 kilometres.
Produced 25,000 cells every second.

All this was achieved without a thought from you,
so cherish and take good care of this cleverness.

CONTENTS

Relax into Health

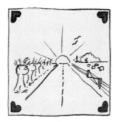

At some point in their lives, most people become aware that life encompasses not only birth, expansion, success, good health, pleasure and prosperity, but also loss, sadness, sickness, struggle, decay, pain and death. This realisation came to me in 1996 at the age of twenty-three, when I awoke from a coma in the intensive care unit of a hospital in London, ten days after passing out in West Africa, and began a long, physically and emotionally exhausting road to recovery.

For an active and healthy adult human, it is a strange, almost fascinating experience to wake up in a dysfunctional mental and physical state. I was partially blind, completely deaf, the skin from my palms peeling off, suffering uncontrolled spastic body movements; I'd lost a third of my body weight, and I had no idea of what year it was or what country I was in. My near-death experience totally altered the lens through which I view the world and my life. Although recovery was a long journey, the intense love and appreciation for this gift called life that I felt has not left me for a single moment since then. Another gift was the basic, timeless keys associated with a healthy mind, body and spirit that eighteen months of a slow and frustrating recovery revealed to me. Within this small book I will share these keys with you.

Luckily, I survived to share my story. At certain times in life it can be helpful to hear another person's story; I hope that what has become apparent to me may also strike a chord with you. Feel free to take what feels right for you and leave what does not. Don't force yourself to do anything; just embrace what resonates with you, try it, then give it some time to settle into your normal daily routine. Just relax and allow your health to sort itself out easily and naturally. Your body is more intelligent than you are led to believe—more, even, than you could ever imagine. Please give the mastery of your own being a chance to prove and express itself with ease.

This book is small so that you can carry it with you, and contains five main sections. They can be read separately or in sequence. Chapter 1 shows the entire health spectrum from optimal health to death, and explains why it is important to act now. Time is ticking by, and your health is being affected! This chapter also discusses the major types of stressors that we are all subject to, as humans tend to deal with similar stressful themes throughout life. Chapter 2 highlights the major models of health and sick care. In it, I also share my journey from a life-threatening situation to embracing a wellness-oriented, vitalistic lifestyle.

Chapter 3 offers alternative solutions to health and sickness. I've titled it "Living the Undoctored Life." It is about self-care and healthcare. Living a healthy life is not rocket science. I have listed suggestions that will guide you into a long-term quality of life. Consistency of effort and long-term thinking are the keys to this chapter.

Chapter 4 examines your deeply held values and beliefs. It has you look at your choices and the decisions you make, whether consciously or subconsciously. These are based on your values. Chapter 5 focuses on what, in my opinion is the easiest, least expensive, and most effective health measure that you can take: drink water! Lastly, the conclusion summarises all the ideas presented and puts them together. Don't skip this part just because it's a summary. You will find that reading it several times is an easy way of letting the information seep in.

You will notice that I return to one key point again and again: the problem is lost health, not acquired sickness. The solution is regaining health, not conquering sickness. Repetition is important. In my opinion, it can take a long time for us to absorb this kind of perspective-changing information, but each time we read or hear it, it sinks in a little deeper.

Some may label me an idealist, and they may be right. Bear in mind, though, that this is a book about healthy and connected living, not merely surviving. Getting and staying healthy is not for the whiners who would rather sit on the sidelines, watch life go by and offer negative comments on topics they know little about. Health is a "hands-on" subject. Lasting health is also counter to the most prevalent social disease of our time: short-term thinking and instant gratification. As a society we have increasingly become victims of fast living: fast cars, fast relationships, fast food, fast diets and fast health fads. In that sense, some of my concepts are idealistic.

Some may question the scientific basis for my assertions. I have a few thoughts on this. First, do we really always need scientific experts to answer our questions for us? Common sense and logic can also play a role. In the case of healthcare, what if "experts" are often actually dispensers of outdated ideas, reliant on flawed sources of information, swayed by conflicting interests? Secondly, most "scientific" studies these days have grossly skewed and dubious outcomes, usually due to their financial implications. Modern science, in my opinion, has taken an almost bizarre view of the human being as unnecessarily complicated, expensive, and machine-like, viewing people as the contents of a test tube that can be "fixed" with chemical compounds. Although these chemicals or medicines may have a lot of science behind them, it is not the type of science that appeals to my logical mind. Scientific research also has limitations. It was only thirty years ago that medical science claimed nutritional or mental problems had nothing to do with disease processes—an awfully outdated view in today's health climate. Fifty years ago, famous medical doctors were promoting cigarettes for relaxation. Furthermore, even when they do turn out to be correct, many scientific theories have taken a long time to prove.

But also, a simple truth that many of us have forgotten is that there is a magical and intangible element in the process of healing and recovery from sickness, which can never be scientifically measured: the role of your body's intelligence, the role of the mind and the impact of unresolved emotions. The intellectual arrogance that "science knows better" frustrates me: the theories as opposed to the experience, the explanations as opposed to the results. There are literally millions of people with "miraculous" recovery stories that cannot be explained by today's science. As a society we tend measure everything. However, not everything is or ever will be measurable for health and healing.

I have tried not to cite too much evidence from other sources to bolster my conclusions. In that sense my work is quite personal. This book is based mostly on my evidence in practice, not evidence-based practice. There are no fast tracks to health or promised miracle cures here. I have simple tools and concepts that help you to understand your body intimately and achieve optimum health—slowly, surely and consistently, in a relaxed and healthy manner.

This is a simple book with timeless keys derived from events that happened to me. These keys are not another new "health fad" or lofty new-age concepts, but are far more important, enduring and substantial. My ideas and views are practical, down to earth, logical—and they work. They may conflict with some of your current ideas concerning health, or may not appeal to you initially. Give them time to sink in. It may even take years for you to understand them—not because they are intellectual, but because they are better understood through doing rather than thinking about them. They will provide you with some new insights around this essential topic of health and give you some practical guidance to help you incorporate healthy living into your daily routine.

Let me be clear that I am in no way targeting or blaming anyone for poor health decisions made in the past. I am no saint: I enjoy a beer with my mates, eat chips with my children, spend too much time on my phone and am sometimes too busy for my own good. In fact, I am continually learning and fine-tuning myself as my understanding of health continues to develop and expand.

I feel that the timing of this book is crucial and important. Here in Singapore, we have one of the most elaborate and expensive healthcare systems of the modern developed world. Billions of *your* dollars get pumped into "research" every year. Yet we have more sick people in Singapore now than ever before—more people suffering from a litany of ailments from cancer, diabetes and depression to hormonal and sexual dysfunction, sleep disturbances and allergies. I think we need to ask why this is so. We need to identify possible answers and get on with logical, affordable solution-based action.

With the ever-increasing costs of caring for sickness, I believe that government efforts to improve "healthcare" are as effective as moving the deck chairs on the Titanic. Of course money needs to be spent on upgrading hospitals and treatments, but simultaneously, money needs to be injected into raising the health of the community, not just treating the sick. I believe that following the advice in this book will not only help your individual health, whatever age you may be, but will also help the greater financial health of the nation. With the aging population, public resources for health will be spread ever thinner. As a result, the use of personal resources and personal control over healthcare decisions will dramatically increase. It's time to reach the summit of health in a natural way. It's time to get back to basic common sense.

So, please, relax into this little book written by me for you. It combines knowledge gained from personal experience, countless books about health, numerous seminars I have attended, and my own observations in private practice as a doctor of chiropractic. I have taken it as my own personal responsibility to introduce a new model of healthcare to the people of Singapore, where the focus is on health, not on disease. I dream of an affordable healthcare system that is friendly both to people and to this beautiful planet, and that supports healthy, high-quality living.

Yours in health,

Vismai

Chapter 1

What Is Health?

If health was sold by the bottle, there would be a shortage of bottles.

—Folk saying

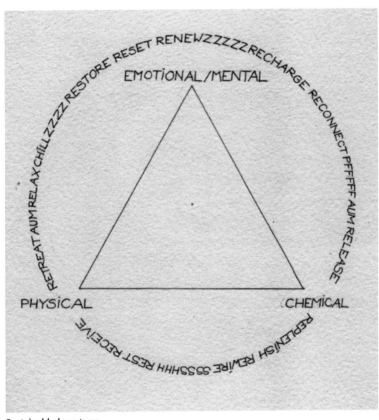

Sustainable long-term
health depends on a
number of interconnected
factors.

Our world has become intensely focused on sickness—not on health. The multi-billion-dollar medical industry is now one of the most lucrative forms of business in the world. Sickness has its own specific language that describes changes to your normal anatomy, with many words such as cancer, diabetes, cardiovascular disease and Alzheimer's disease entering our everyday vocabulary. When your body is not sick, it is generally characterised with one word: normal. Apparently the abnormal (as opposed to the normal) situation is easier to see, prove and experience. But "normal," as we will see later, also has many variations.

When we get sick, the problem has little to do with the sickness itself. The problem lies with lost health, not with acquired sickness. I believe the lasting solution lies not with fighting sickness and disease, but by improving and regaining health. It's like considering the glass half full as opposed to half empty. This different perspective is important.

When we are in a healthy state, we have more energy for our family members, we sleep better, we're able to handle work-related stress with greater ease. Body weight and sexual function are more balanced. Our potential to earn a good income is greater. All of these things are at stake when your body is not functioning well.

Sickness is the absence of health

Let's consider for a moment why our world is so focused on sickness.

> Science acknowledges what is objective (factual) and what is
> subjective (non-factual). However, it always focuses on the objective
> facts. For example, sound is a fact. If we want to make sound, we can
> clap our hands, we can scream, or turn on some music. Silence, on
> the other hand, is a lack of sound; it is subjective. The best examples
> are light and darkness. Light is factual: we can light a match, turn on
> a lamp. Darkness is subjective, existing only when there is no source
> of light. Light is measured in watts; darkness, on the other hand,
> is immeasurable. If there is light, what has happened to darkness?
> Darkness does not crawl into a corner or slip out through a crack
> under the door. Darkness can be considered infinite, immeasurable,
> or abysmal without light. When you are not sick, health is present.
> It is seemingly immeasurable, or described as normal. The pull
> to focus on better health is less urgent than the emergency that
> sickness presents. Health does not exist as a measurable thing. All the
> darkness of the world cannot harm the light from a candle.
> —Joseph B. Strauss, *Enhance Your Life Experience*

So science focuses on objective facts. When medical science started
researching health and disease, the choice was made to consider
sickness as objective, or factual, and health as subjective, unreal—
probably because the characteristics of disease stand out more than
the characteristics of health, just as light stands out from darkness.
Everything that deviates from "normal" stands out more. Imagine
the implications if we had chosen health, not sickness, as the basis for

centuries of medical study? In fact, the alternative healthcare paradigm has done just that, for hundreds of years. Choosing health as the focus is a comprehensive and simple answer to the unnecessary complications and expenses that dominate modern sick care.

The irony is that, until recently, health measurements have often been criticised as being unscientific by the science-based medical establishment. This may be because during a typical medical undergraduate programme, little time is spent studying health; the focus is on sickness. In contrast, during my five-year chiropractic degree, at least 50 percent of the time was spent studying health. Luckily for all of us, smart technology offers precise tools to measure your health. Technology can now measure tendencies in your body (heart rate variability, blood sugar levels, the sleep-wake cycle) that provide objective feedback on how your body is functioning. Tracking and acting on this data allows you to change your lifestyle long before you get a disease.

The elements of health

Sustainable, long-term health depends on four interconnected factors:

Physical—the body's structural system. This includes all the muscles, bones, tendons, nerves, blood vessels and organs. A body with poor structural integrity can experience aches and pains, poor sleep and fatigue. These may in fact contribute to all disease processes.

Chemical—the biochemical and physiological processes. These include the absorption and utilisation of nutrients, the excretion of toxins, the intracellular functions and the body's use of water.

Emotional—The mind, emotions and spirit. We all know these things play an enormous role in health, but they are often deeply private, personal and immeasurable. As Hippocrates (460–377 BCE) said, "It is more important to know what sort of person has a disease than to know what sort of disease a person has."

Rest—We all need rest; taking a break gives your mind and body time to regenerate. Make this a priority; as people sometimes say, "Actively pursue relaxation." Rest gives resilience during your workday. Hippocrates also puts it nicely: "Doing nothing is sometimes a good remedy."

The human being is a complex organism. In any organism, health is normal; if signs of a lack of health emerge, it is noticed. We take a healthy body for granted: when we go to bed, we do not think, "My kidneys produced urine so well today," or "My pancreas adjusted my blood sugar so smoothly this afternoon." We only act when these things do not work any more. At that point we stumble on the problems, frustrations, and misunderstanding of the modern medical system. This model focuses on treating the signs of lost health, on fighting symptoms more than re-establishing and recovering that health. It pushes us to deal with situations when they become urgent. This needs to change. In only dealing with problems when they have become emergencies, life becomes a short-term, expensive, problem-solving, vulnerable experience, especially when it comes to your health.

Focus on health

We know for a fact that 80 percent of people get back pain. This means there is a big chance that you will get it, too. Why not start taking care of your spine right now? Exercise it. Develop a solid muscular core in your body. Move your spine while you are at work, especially if you sit behind a computer. Why wait until the inevitable pain comes and you need to seek emergency care for it?

Let's relax and ease into these ideas regarding health and make them a part of your everyday life. The reality is that sometimes we are sick and sometimes we are not. Sometimes we have a lot of energy and other times we are tired. Sometimes you can take on the entire world, at other times the smallest irritant sends you mad. Health and sickness are part of the same single process that starts when you are born and ends when you die. There will always be good and bad days, weeks, months and years.

The full spectrum of health

Let's take a wider view of health, broadening the tunnel-vision view of sickness. Looking at the full spectrum of health will give us a more realistic and all-encompassing perspective on how real health works throughout the lifetime of a human. By doing this we gain an overall picture of how our sickness and health blend together. If health and sickness are viewed as a continuum, "life" stands at one end and "death" stands at the other. That continuum can be divided into five phases. I'll call the first two phases "wellness areas." The third phase is neutral; the fourth and fifth are "sickness areas."

Phase one

In the first phase, you feel just fine, and your body functions perfectly: your liver filters your blood, your kidneys excrete waste, and your pancreas regulates your blood-sugar levels. Your heartbeat is regular and your breathing smooth. You feel energetic and your spirit is bright. Your skin and hair have a healthy glow, your eyes are clear, and you have a youthful presence, no matter how old you are. You can easily adapt to different environments because your body's senses are working well. You can touch, hear, smell, taste, and see with great detail. Your body has an ideal balance of strength and flexibility, and your weight is proportional to your height. Your body and breath have little odor. You have two to three bowel movements per day, so your body gets rid of toxins quickly and with ease. You deal with emotions quickly and do not bottle up mental problems. You fall asleep easily; your sleep regenerates your body and is of a peaceful nature. You have a healthy sexual function. Your body's general pH is alkaline in nature. You have had healthy lifestyle tendencies for a long time, hydrating your body well and taking in a good natural diet. You are well grounded in reality. You have long-term ideas about your health.

Phase two

In the second phase, you also feel good. A symptom may emerge occasionally, but it will disappear without effort. If you focus on the four pillars of health, you can return to phase one. Your short-term lost health can be explained easily; for example, you caught a cold because you didn't get enough sleep. Your bodily functions work less smoothly than in phase one, but you may not notice it. The changes are too subtle to experience as symptoms. This phase is like a car that needs an oil change to run more smoothly—something the driver does not really notice. Although you have had healthy tendencies for a long time, the aging process may be catching up with you. The accumulation of toxins over the years may be silently changing your body. For example, that accident you had fifteen years ago will finally start causing you pain, and the changes are clearly visible on an X-ray.

Phase three

I characterise the third, neutral phase as an early departure from wellness. Most people are actually functioning in this phase. The tricky thing is that there are often no clear symptoms, especially in people under the age of forty. There may be recurring symptoms, but nothing urgent. It is much more difficult to return to the full wellness of phase one or two from this state, but it's still far from the acute fifth phase. Blood test results are generally normal in this phase. However, unresolved emotions are beginning to pile up at a cellular level because the stress of life accumulates over time. The body's pH may be more acidic now, allowing disease processes to gain momentum. You no longer feel energetic, but you are not lethargic either. While you may not feel depressed, you are not as happy as you were in the earlier phases. Your body odors are becoming stronger. Your eyes are beginning to develop black spots in them. Your skin becomes dry and dull because your body is less hydrated than it used to be.

Phase four

In the fourth phase, symptoms begin to take on more momentum in their development, and certain functions are lost. However, there is no clear pathology; your doctor may be unable to give you a clear diagnosis. People in phase four may have several vague complaints—persistent stomachache, fatigue, inability to concentrate, aches and pains. You'll say "I just can't get through the day like I used to." You find it difficult to lose weight or you gain weight easily, and your body changes shape as it accumulates fat—largely due to the accumulation of toxins over time. You often need a holiday or a break from work. Stress may increase, be it family- or work-related. Most people have a tendency to look outside themselves for reasons why life is not as easy as they wish it were: spouse, job, studies, bank balance. If you are chronically tired, you blame it on your work. If you are poor, you blame it on the government. If you are overweight, you blame it on hormones, fast food, or your genes.

A person may spend several years in phase four. This is a phase where people often push themselves against what their body is telling them. Most people in this phase realise that they are becoming sick, but they simply don't bother to acknowledge it. Without taking drastic measures at this stage, chronic sickness and disease are inevitable.

Phase five

The fifth phase presents clear symptoms that are connected with a certain disease. Objective findings are measurable in your blood, and can be diagnosed through physical examination or X-ray images. You may be told you have cancer, osteoarthritis, osteoporosis, depression or cardiovascular disease. At this point, you may feel relieved to finally "know" what is wrong with you. Unfortunately, you are comforted by having a medical diagnosis and knowing that specific treatment can begin from this point on. At last, you can explain clearly why you have been feeling so terrible for the last few months or years.

From my perspective, these diseases are merely a manifestation of health being reduced to dangerous levels. Instead of focusing on restoring that health, most people chose to fill their bodies with poison in the form of medicine. Instead of choosing to optimise their health, most people will opt to fight disease. Remember, the major problem is not the onset of disease, it is the loss of health. Unresolved emotions may have in fact made such vibrational changes at the cellular level that your cells appear cancerous. Your sweat becomes metallic because the body is chronically stressed and has an acidic pH. In phase five, a prognosis is estimated for your disease: you are in an emergency state of sickness.

The diagnosis you receive in phase five has to begin its manifestation somewhere. This is usually in phase two, and often takes years to develop to the point that you reach phase five. Remember, your liver is not suddenly full of cancer; your pancreas does not suddenly stop producing insulin; you do not suddenly get fat; you do not suddenly become burnt out. The truth is that you develop your diagnosis over time.

A good example is spinal degeneration, because we all suffer from it, and it is a downhill process. It is often diagnosed later in life—after the age of fifty—by an X-ray image. However, the degeneration process actually begins twenty to thirty years before it can be seen clearly in an X-ray. Early signs include a decreased range of motion in the neck and low back, chronic stiffness, postural changes like rounded shoulders, a forward-leaning head and neck, uneven ear levels, uneven leg lengths and back pain. Your sleep may suffer because you cannot get comfortable. Your fingers might begin to tingle because you are slowly losing your natural neck curve and the nerves become chronically irritated.

Although wellness and sickness are sometimes not as clear-cut as the above explanation makes them, viewing your health as a spectrum of overlapping phases is easier to grasp than one-word explanations such as "normal" or "unwell."

Homeostasis

A trauma such as a car accident can cause someone to jump from phase one to phase five suddenly. This is an exceptional situation, however. What usually happens is that the transition between phases is so gradual as to go unnoticed. Furthermore, the phases may overlap. The slow buildup can be seen in remarks like, "I used to get through the work week easily, but now I'm wiped out by Wednesday," and "I don't win at squash like I used to—I guess I'm not twenty any more." Very slowly, your body starts to refuse to do what you want it to. This is not *disease*, but I would call it *dis*-ease, as opposed to *with*-ease.

Think of a mother who has just had her third child: she gets tired more easily, has less patience; her neck and shoulders often hurt from heavy lifting and breastfeeding. Or think of a man who used to be able to work at his computer for five hours at a clip, but now has to get up every half-hour to stretch. His concentration is easily broken and he makes more errors. Or what about the chiropractor who spends all day bending over a table? His spine is straight as an arrow when he's twenty-five, but by the time he is forty-five his shoulders are far more rounded. The people in these examples may say, "I don't want to complain," or "I'm going to stop whining and move on." This attitude sets a solid base for more dangerous disease processes to build up into the long term, ten to twenty years from now. Stress must be balanced in the long term.

Now I'll offer a word for you to consider: homeostasis. My wellness model, like the modern medical industry, has its own language. Some of the words will be familiar to you, but they tend to be more subjective and open to interpretation. Terms like "wellness," "anti-aging," and even the word "health" itself are all open-ended, individualistic words. They are not black-and-white. In my experience, however, the words used in my wellness model are strongly connected to the most common real-life situations. They encompass the entire health spectrum—not just conditions occurring in phase five that are described in medical-industry terms. Understand that only perhaps 10 percent of us have a diagnosis that places us clearly into phase five. The other 90 percent of us are simply considered normal or healthy, regardless of where we are on the rest of the spectrum.

Homeostasis is one of the most essential concepts you will encounter in this book. This term relates to the need for balance and adaptation; that is, processing the signals from the body and taking the necessary action to help support it. Failure to do this inevitably leads to *dis*-ease. So when embracing all this health advice, be sure to stay connected, feel and listen to your body's needs. Modify your ideas as your body gives you feedback—in other words, ease into it. Be aware, conscious and mindful.

Homeostasis is what happens when you realise a need for balance and adapt your actions to recover that balance when it is disturbed. A simple example is putting on a coat before going out into the cold: You don't think twice about dressing warmly for the weather; your body tells you that you need to do it. Another example with the same adaptive theme but a reverse outcome would be a man in his mid-forties, seemingly at the peak of his life—never smokes, drinks only socially, is happily married with healthy children, has a successful but busy career—who suffers a heart attack and dies one day when he is jogging. This is an example of a man who either does not hear or chooses to push through the warning signals that his body gives him. For 40 percent of people who suffer a heart attack, death is their first warning sign.

The way you feel may not be represented by how you function. You should be honest with yourself when you know that you have been doing too much for too long. Respect your limitations, take the necessary action steps and give your body some time to heal. Do this in phase one, two, or three—long before the continued stress has the time to develop a disease in your body. I worked in Amsterdam, New York, Tasmania and Jakarta before coming to work in Singapore. I've put my hands on very busy people, and I can feel this stress deeply embedded in their bodies when I touch them.

The path back to health

As we've established, disease emerges when one's health breaks down to dangerous levels. Again, the problem is not that disease is acquired, it is that health is lost. So how does your health break down, and how can you regain it?

This single question is essential, because it points you in the direction of your health, not your disease. It puts you in control of your recovery rather than a doctor or drug. "How did I lose my health?" is a more empowering question than "How did I contract this disease?" because it forces you to look inside instead of outside for your answers. It allows you to trust your body's innate healing mechanism. When you honestly ask yourself this question, answers will be revealed.

Asking, "I have this disease; how can I treat it?" puts the focus on the disease. It forces you to search for someone who specialises in your disease, not a wellness practitioner who is interested in restoring your health. The specialist deals with your disease: all day, every day; the focus is not on present or future health. You search for known medicine for your disease, a specific drug for your specific sickness. You swallow, inject or inhale this medicine religiously, no questions asked. You do this without considering the poisons in the medicine because you want to treat your disease, not your health. Your overall health, from this perspective, is less important than the acquired disease. You'll deal with your lost health later; you just want to get rid of the disease.

There are some pervasive examples of such an "outside-in" view of health in our society. For example, the belief that cats cause allergies, that medicine will make you healthy or fix the cause of a health problem, that the common cold is caused by a virus—all these are assumptions that are cast in doubt by the ideas in this book. If the beliefs just described are yours, some of what follows in the next chapters may upset or frustrate you. Your model of health might be quite different from mine. That's totally OK! You may view life as an outside-in rather than an inside-out experience. If you have no interest in changing this perspective, I wish you success in pursuing health. If you're curious, however, I invite you to read on and keep an open mind. Take what you like and leave what you don't. I think you'll find it worth your time.

Chapter 2

Models of Healthcare

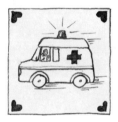

The greatest of follies is to sacrifice health for any other advantage.

—Arthur Schopenhauer, philosopher

AND LIFT, AND DON'T EVEN DO CARDIO. IT'S BAD F(
JOINTS. ALSO, DON'T EAT TOO MUCH PROTEIN AND
E SURE YOU'RE SLEEPING A LOT. BUT DON'T BE SEDE
Y. BUT DON'T BE TOO ACTIVE, IT'S BAD FOR YOUR BL(
SSURE. MAKE SURE YOU REPLACE ALL YOUR LOST SAL
NEVER EAT TOO MUCH SODIUM. IT'S EASY. JUST EAT V
.ES. DON'T EAT POTATOES THOUGH OR CORN. FRUIT I
OUSLY GOOD FOR YOU, AND ALSO IT'S ALL SUGAR ANI
) FOR YOU. SUGAR, I FORGOT TO MENTION, IS A VITAL
RCE OF QUICK BURNING CARB(S THAT YOUR
IN NEEDS TO SURVIVE. AN   ) AVOID IT /
COSTS. PROTEIN IS   'S. MAKE SU
EAT A LOT OF IT.   STARVE YO
F UNLESS YOU'RE   STING
) THAN IT'S OKAY T(B
'T OVER HYDRATE. BEIN
LTHIEST LIFESTYLE, AN
3VIOUSLY SUPER GOOD
CURY AND KILLING YOU.
' FOR VITAMIN D AND S

Are you confused about what is good for you? If you are, it's no wonder, since the information coming at you from all directions is completely contradictory.

Are you confused about what is good for you? If you are, it's no wonder, since the information coming at you from all directions is completely contradictory.

In this chapter I will talk about models of healthcare. The word "model" means a way of thinking combined with action. It is a combination of visions, missions, action pathways and end results. All models of thought—from sports to business, from religion to healthcare—have their strengths and weaknesses. They also have their own subjective interpretation, and they need to be reviewed from time to time to see if they are still relevant and useful. For example, tactics that were used by the world's best football players thirty years ago probably don't work in today's fast-paced, highly skilled competition. Sure, there are skills that are timeless, but many of the approaches considered essential back then are of no use in the game today.

How does this apply to health? After years of deep contemplation, I have concluded that there are three vastly different models at work in our current health- and sickness-care system:

- Emergency healthcare
- Rehabilitation and maintenance
- Wellness care

Whichever model you adhere to—consciously or unconsciously—has a tremendous impact on how you react to health advice. Furthermore, each of these three very different models of healthcare must be available to us. This is because health needs vary depending on age, accidents, ongoing stress levels, and so on. Sometimes there are emergencies in your health that need short-term immediate attention. Or you may need to pay extra attention to some aspect of your health to achieve a goal—trying to improve your balance and coordination as you train to run a marathon, for example. At some point you may break your leg, or find yourself in the middle of a divorce or other crisis that causes you to need regular bodywork to help you relax and sleep.

Different health requirements are served differently by the three care models. The key is to know which model to choose and when to choose it. Choosing the wrong model at the wrong time is like trying to fit a square peg into a round hole. It can be done, but not without unnecessary struggle.

Emergency healthcare: the first model

To give a real-life example of the different models at work, I will share my own story with you. I was extremely fortunate to have all models of sickness and healthcare available to me through a health crisis. I am alive because the emergency medical model saved me from imminent death.

It was mid-March, 1996, around 7 AM. My travel companion, Bernie, and I were somewhere between Accra and Cape Coast in Ghana, West Africa. I awoke with a faint headache but I could feel it rapidly increasing in intensity. My blood felt warm, and I was desperately thirsty. For some intuitive reason I knew I was about to get extremely sick very quickly. I shook Bernie awake: "Bernie, mate! We've got to get out of here now!

Take me to the hospital in Accra!" (In Accra, I could go to Northridge Hospital, the hospital for foreigners and upper-class locals.) I begged him to get me some water. But he couldn't find drinking water for me anywhere. I have never needed water with such urgency in my life. Just before we arrived at the bus stop, I began to hallucinate: when I looked at the ground I could only see the sky, and it was spinning like a merry-go-round. I was disoriented, drowsy, and going in and out of consciousness.

We thought we would find water at the bus station, but there wasn't any. I let out a cry of despair, feeling myself losing my mind because I needed water so badly. I smashed the side of the bus with such force that I thought I'd broken my hand. Within a short time—though it felt like an eternity—water arrived. Some Ghanaian men at that bus stop cared for me like I was their son. They held me upright and they poured water all over me. I quickly drank about three litres and the hallucinations became less intense.

We arrived in Accra, and as I stepped down from the bus the noise, dust, loud strange language, barking dogs and thick air pollution all got the better of me, and I collapsed. I was in a bad state. I was in an emergency. I needed a doctor who knew everything about sickness. I needed help from outside because my body was failing me on the inside. I found myself in model one: emergency healthcare. Luckily for me, this model exists; it saved my life. It can save yours, too.

This model requires quick, accurate short-term thinking and utilises diagnostic tools and instruments. In the emergency healthcare model, the right decisions save lives and the wrong ones cost lives: rigid protocols are used to reduce the risk of human error. It has its own vocabulary and style of questioning—very specific and to the point. My friend Bernie had several questions for the staff at the hospital: "Will my friend die, or is he going to survive? Can you help him, or will he have to leave the country to seek better specialists? What is the diagnosis? Will there be permanent physical or mental damage?"

Bernie slept in my room at Northridge Hospital. My hallucinations had become so intense that my grasp of reality was slowly leaving me, but I do retain a few impressions of that time before I was put on a plane to an intensive-care facility in England. One was being given the "anointing of the sick." The people of Ghana are deeply Christian, and this is the sacrament given to Christians just before they die. Having been raised in a Catholic family, I knew this was significant, and I realised how near death I was. This first glimpse at the possibility of dying gave me a deep longing to see my family and friends. As I waited on the airport tarmac on a stretcher waiting to be flown to London for treatment, I remember Bernie wishing me luck in heaven, saying, "You really deserve to go there!" Those were his farewell words to me.

The Ghanaian doctor accompanied me on that emergency flight and he was one of the first people I saw when I woke up in London. Although I have no memories of the flight itself, I know the airplane was filled with the kind of essential medical equipment that characterises the emergency-care model—things like antibiotics to keep infection at bay; an intravenous drip; a heart monitor; a defibrillator in case my heart stopped; protocols to keep track of my heartbeat, respiratory rate, urine output, conscious state and temperature; and extremely sterile equipment for the doctor to use. As in many emergency situations, time was going to be crucial to my outcome.

I came to slowly in a bright, white, clean room—too orderly and sterile to be in Africa, but I had no idea where I was or even what year it was. My surroundings were ultramodern, as if I had woken up in the far future. The atmosphere felt foggy, hazy and cloudlike, almost dreamy; I tried to speak but only unintelligible babble came out. I couldn't hear anything, either, but I felt my mouth and tongue moving awkwardly.

I looked out the window and saw the doctors looking in at me. They gave an impression of sterility and authority; there was a futuristic vibe about them. Doctors who work in the emergency model are specialists, and they wear clothes that represent authority, like the classic white medical coat. You can tell by the way people treat them that they are in charge. As my hearing returned, I could hear them speaking, and even their tone of voice had an authoritative ring. They were looking at me like I was some kind of prehistoric dinosaur. A nurse came into my room wearing a spacesuit; in the absence of a specific diagnosis, I was in quarantine. They knew that I had malaria, pneumonia and hepatitis A, but the other part of my sickness was unclear. They could see it in my blood, but they had no known name for it, and to this day it remains undiagnosed. Later the doctors told me that I had initially been flown to one hospital but was rejected for admission. They put me in a helicopter, and then flew me to St. George's in Tooting, London, one of the largest hospitals in Europe. My vital signs showed I was in complete survival mode: my resting heart rate was racing at 140 beats per minute—three times faster than normal; my breathing was fast and very shallow because only the top lobe of my left lung was working, and my body temperature was a dangerous 40 degrees Celsius. I was fighting to survive.

Life in intensive care at St. George's quickly became exhausting. Having to pee into a catheter, poo into a tube, and be fed through a tube in my nose was painful and tiresome. I had a tight mask around my nose to supply oxygen which, after a few days, felt like a thin metal rod squeezing into my skin.

I will always be indebted to the knowledge, professionalism, seriousness, commitment, love and teamwork that the intensive care staff so carefully bestowed on me. I could feel their years of knowledge and experience. I knew I was in the best possible place to have any chance of survival. But the fundamental nature of the intensive-care unit is that death is often close by, no matter how skilled your doctors are. After a few days of relative stability, all my vital signs started failing. Doctors came rushing in, and I could tell by the concerned looks on their faces that I was likely facing my last few hours of life. But I was too tired to go on any more.

For me, the end of my short but beautiful life was OK—I felt peaceful, even grateful with my imminent death staring at me. That was such an intense moment of total surrender and acceptance. My Australian nurse, Karen, came to me with a piece of paper to write down some last words I wanted to say. I was totally at peace with the fact that it was time to die. I was full of love and gratitude for every single person I had ever met, for every single thing I had ever done: it was bliss. For me, there was certainly no struggle with surrendering to my death.

However, I was still emotionally attached to my life. Reminiscences and reflections kept flashing into my head. The fact that my father and brother were on a refueling stop in Singapore on their way over from Australia to be with me motivated me to hang on and see them one last time. As a last-ditch effort I decided to meditate, whatever that was. I had no friends who meditated and I had no training in it. For me, only new-age hippies did that strange stuff. But I meditated, for the first time in my life.

(As a side note, I recommend meditation to anybody who is interested. These days, the one addiction I have in my life is meditation, because it's a fast-track way of connecting with my inner self or the source that created me. Meditation, prayer, or mindfulness connects you to the same power that made your body—which is the same power that heals your body.)

In any event, my heart stopped and I found myself at one hell of a changing point. I was having a near-death experience. It was exactly how you hear about it: the tunnel of white light, my life being played to me like an overly detailed short film, so much love it was almost painful, intense gratitude for human life and no linear time or space. The whole kit and caboodle: I was in heaven. (For a full account of my experience, see the Appendix on page 121.) I woke up fighting for my life again, but this time it was different. Inside, I knew I had been to rock bottom, and from that point on I would recover. My silent, teary father had arrived, and he refused to let go of my hand. My jet-lagged brother lay asleep in the chair in the corner of my room. The arrival of my family gave me a boost of support and energy that no medicine could ever have provided.

At length, my hearing returned. The first sound I heard was the nurse taking off her rubber gloves and washing her hands. Then there was the sucking and pumping noise of the machine next to the bed which delivered liquidised food into my stomach via a tube in my nose. The constant racket was irritating, but it was better than being deaf. I began to be able to see again. The life-support machine had significantly raised my blood pressure, bursting the small arteries in my eyes and causing countless blind spots in my vision. It was as if I was viewing everything through a block of Swiss cheese.

Then I was able to eat again. The first thing I ate was vanilla ice cream, which tasted absolutely delicious; I felt as though I hadn't eaten in months. Then I was able to sit up again. The physiotherapists had to help me reach a sitting posture, but the fact that I was no longer lying on my back was promising. And then I was able to walk again. I had lost so much weight that my knees were the fattest part of my body. Walking just a few steps made me laugh and cry at the same time. On the one hand I was terribly excited that I was walking again, yet on the other hand I felt appalled at the reality of my situation. Since my condition had deteriorated so rapidly, it was as if I needed extra time to mentally accept that I could not walk normally. I would look down at my legs and see that they were simply not working properly. They struggled do what my brain was telling them.

Rehabilitation and maintenance: the second model

Time went by and I kept improving in small, regular increments. I was transferred from the intensive-care unit to a normal hospital ward. My first shower there was a scary experience—similar, I imagine, to what older people experience when their bodies start to fail them. I didn't dare walk over the shower step. I had to summon all my arm strength to turn the light on, and I didn't have the power to turn the tap on or off. The staff in the ward were not as vigilant as they had been in intensive care, so I was stuck in that shower for what seemed like hours. But I managed. I had entered the next model of sick care: rehabilitation and maintenance.

My body wanted to get better. I could sense its efforts to renew. I felt hungry, thirsty, tired and determined, sensations that had been absent in the previous months. I was back in touch with my homeostatic mechanism (see page 23). Another secret revealed itself here: I realised that my body knew the way back to health. I felt a deep sense of peaceful assurance that I would be OK. I had been in a sort of whirling soup the past few months and I had had no control over how I would respond or adapt to my environment. Constant exhaustion was now replaced by a less intense daily phase of tiredness. Automatic feeding by a tube in my nose was punctuated by moments of hunger. Instead of receiving fluids through a drip in my arm, I drank vitamin- and mineral-infused drinks from a carton—astronaut food, they told me.

Time plays an important role in maintenance, but in this model it is not a matter of life and death: the role of time is more predictable. For example, if you break your arm, it will take approximately eight weeks for your bone to heal, depending on the type of fracture. If you bruise your ribs, it takes about six weeks for your body to do its repair work. Following a hip replacement operation, it may be six months before you feel completely recovered. After a heart bypass operation or cancer treatment you may be tired for up to twelve months.

In this model you are typically in touch with your circumstances, and you take a more active role in the repair process. You are no longer dependent on machines to keep you alive. Most people show interest in getting better, and other less urgent, less specific types of questions arise: "What can I do at home to help the recovery process?" "What can I do to minimise this happening again?" "When will I be able to return to work?" "Will physical activity help my recovery?"

This model is less black and white than the emergency model, but you still have clear symptoms. You have a "sick story" to tell your friends and family. This model focuses on individual body parts: your hip, shoulder, eyes, heart. Equipment characteristically used in this model includes a walking stick or crutches for support; supporting braces—a knee brace, a low-back support belt; supportive tape like that used after a shoulder dislocation; exercise equipment used under the guidance of a trained physiotherapist; special creams or ointments to speed healing of injured skin. Medicines commonly used in this model are the more non-specific, general types: pain relief medication, muscle relaxants, "feel-good" placebo medication, general antibiotics.

From the perspective of a chiropractor and health and wellness promoter, this model is frustrating. Most people—those who live by ideas like "Stop whining and move on," or "No pain, no gain"—stop treatment when the pain disappears, because they no longer perceive sickness. This attitude has its short-term advantages, in that you don't panic about every little pain you feel, but long-term disadvantages in that you often ignore what your body is telling you, and sooner or later it will catch up with you. Symptoms are often the last thing to appear in a sickness process and often the first thing to leave once the treatment begins.

In any event, I was finally able to leave the hospital with my father and brother. My senses were overwhelmed by the world outside after living at the hospital for months. Leaving those rotating doors of St. George's Hospital was, in a funny way, like returning to life after my near-death experience, offering sudden insights. My first whiff of the air outside the hospital was full of secondhand cigarette smoke. The hospital entrance was surrounded by patients in wheelchairs, patients standing with a drip attached to their arms, and even patients on hospital beds—all smoking, smoking like they couldn't get enough of it. (Interestingly enough, some of my favourite clients smoke. They often describe the act of having a smoke as "having a little moment with myself.")

One of those classic black London cabs took us back to where my father and brother were staying. I saw an old man struggling to exit a telephone box during the ride home and I fully understood why he couldn't get out; I had a new appreciation for his physical predicament and vulnerability in what seemed to me an excessively fast-paced city lifestyle. Bless him.

I was classified as an outpatient. Three times a week I reported to the doctors specializing in different body parts at the hospital, but essentially my body itself and time did the healing. I was no longer taking prescription medicine. The most worrying aspect for me at that stage was my vision. The large blind spots in my visual field were gone, but straight lines appeared wiggly to me. The eye specialist reassured me that the wiggly vision would leave of its own accord without any need for treatment as time played its natural role.

That eye specialist knew almost everything there was to know about the human eye. I felt reassured by this, because I had questions about my eyes, and he could answer every single one of them. During one of my consultations, I asked him about my hair loss: "When will my hair return to normal?" He replied, "I know nothing about hair." This surprised me at the time, because up until then he had been able to answer all my questions clearly and easily. He said, "First you'll have to go to your doctor and get a referral letter to go to the dermatologist."

"OK," I said. "Do you have a colleague you could recommend?"

"No, dermatology is another department and I've never spoken to any of the dermatologists. But you'll be in good hands," he reassured me.

His answer to this question raised several others for me. Who should I go to? What doctor would be my best bet for getting the right answer to my question? If my hair loss was due to a hair problem, then the dermatologist was the obvious specialist to help me. Or maybe it was due to my poor nutritional and mineral status, and in that case a nutritionist would be my chosen specialist. But they did not talk with one another. How would I know what to do?

This is a classic example of how the maintenance model views the body in separate parts. Specialists such as cardiologists, rheumatologists, neurologists, dermatologists, and so on have clearly delineated boundaries, and maintain almost no contact with one another. They are extremely fixated on the outcomes of blood tests, CT and MRI scans, ECG readings, hair mineral analysis, and other very specific tests. Specialists in this model seem to have an elevated social status in their community. People tend to respect their knowledge.

Wellness care: the third model

Sickness is a situation in which you find out who your real friends are. People that you thought were your friends may disappear, while total strangers step up to bat for you. For me, there were the Ghanaian men at the bus stop and my Aussie nurse, Karen. Then there were Cameron and Sally, whom I had never met before I landed at St. George's. Cam was the brother of a guy that I had lived with for a short time while studying chiropractic. I happened to have their telephone number on the inside of my diary, scribbled on a yellow sticky note. When I arrived in London, the doctors phoned them.

"Do you know this guy?" they asked.

"We've heard of him," they said. "What's the problem? Is there anything we can do to help him?"

The first time I met Cam and Sally they had signed some forms to be my next of kin—the people who made decisions for me because I was incapable of doing so, since I was dying—because my father had not arrived in London yet. Cameron, loving husband of Sally, is a father, a wellness chiropractor and, at the time of this story, the owner of an extremely small apartment in Putney, London. We had never met before, yet they housed my family. I come from a relatively poor family, so the neigbours lent my father some money on short notice to enable him and my brother to come to London and help me get out of the mess I had gotten into. The kindness of strangers was what kept me alive. Before I knew it, I was ready to fly home to Australia. The return visits to my specialists ended and there was no real reason to remain in London any longer. Besides, I just wanted to get home to my mother, sister and friends, so that I could return to some form of "normal" living.

The rehabilitation model can last weeks, months, or years. I was in it for about eighteen months. It took my body a long time to return to its pre-sickness standards. I struggled to put on weight. My muscle strength was appallingly poor: I was so weak that I could not even flick on a light switch, so my parents bought me one of those touch lamps. It took twelve months for my hair to come back. My breath smelled foul for at least six months. I was so extremely tired for at least a year; I just needed to sleep, sleep, and sleep. During this time, my sleep was very deep, because my body was busy recovering twenty-four hours a day.

Mentally, I was confused. I had no interest in people or activities that had once been a big part of my life. Looking back on that time, it was very lonely and depressing for me. There was no drama in this phase of my return to health, because I did not care about anything enough to make it a drama. I simply could not settle back into my old life. Friends came around to visit, but I showed no interest.

As sure as a river inevitably flows to the ocean, though, my recovery gained momentum. Coming from such a low point in my health, I found it easy to feel, see and measure the progress my body was so naturally making, month in month out. Signs characterizing the wellness model of health became a part of my life and personal interest.

The wellness model has its own unique characteristics that set it apart from the first and second models.

- The person is no longer seen as a patient with a sickness to defeat, but rather as a human being with their health levels raised.
- There is a long-term, consistent commitment to pursuing a healthy lifestyle.
- The focus is not on sickness, but on health and optimal functioning.
- There is a humanistic attitude that encourages the development of a friendly relationship with your body. People in this model have a good, clear connection with their body.
- There is interest in good health—not only in preventing or recovering from sickness.
- Physical and mental stress are dealt with more easily than in the previous models.
- When a person does get sick, it is understood from a perspective of lost health more than from a perspective of disease.
- The body is seen as a holistic structure whose parts comprise the whole, rather than being viewed as separate components as in model two. Each system in the body is interconnected with and interdependent upon all other systems in the body.
- Health-related goals are often seen in this model: training to run or walk a marathon, regular attendance at the gym or yoga class, sufficient water consumption. Even in the absence of symptoms, a body assessment may be done to maintain balance and equilibrium. A proactive attitude encourages people to take responsibility for their own health.
- Healthcare practitioners are viewed as partners in the goal of

optimizing health. The therapist is not seen as an authority figure, but more like a normal person with a great set of skills—in contrast to the emergency model, where the treating doctor is definitely an authority figure.

- This model embraces progress, not necessarily perfection.

Adopting the wellness model is about making the quality of your life a priority. "It's not the hours you put in that count, it's what you put into the hours." This model embraces the advanced scientific study of human health, as opposed to human sickness.

It is ironic that we often need some type of crisis for us to appreciate what we have, be it healthy children, a good bank balance, a roof over our heads, food on the table, a mind that works clearly, a peaceful social group or a healthy relationship with our life partner. We so often take what we have for granted until it is gone. I had been to the horrible depths of sickness and I wanted to cherish my body, to care for it like a rare jewel. It was a feeling that rose from within me, not because the doctors told me that I had to take better care of myself, but because I wanted to do it.

My body was a lot more sensitive to my environment than before. The smallest physical, emotional, chemical or spiritual stressors threw me off balance very easily. After not eating for a few months, I could taste chemicals in any food that was not organic. For example, I could no longer taste meat, only the hormones and the drugs taken by the animal whose flesh I was eating. It tasted like poison; I felt that drinking petrol would have been more palatable and not much worse for my health. I know this might sound rather extreme, but my senses were very acute at that point.

In the wellness model you are ahead of the eight ball. Thus, the questions associated with this model come from a different place.

- How can I best care for my body over the long term so that it will deal with moments of stress with greater ease?
- What is the most effective way for me to mentally detoxify myself in stressful phases?
- What is my ideal body weight in relation to my height? If I could achieve this weight, would the joints in my body and the discs in my lower back work more effectively and for a longer time?
- How can I keep my liver and kidneys clean so they can best filter my blood?
- How can I stay in contact with my body so that I can best listen and respond to its needs?
- How can I keep the physical frame of my body balanced and in a perfect level of tension?

From a grassroots perspective, alternative medicine is more cost-effective in the long run than paying rising ever-less-affordable healthcare costs. Yet almost all medical funding and your donation dollars go into study of the current Western medical model that focuses on the cure for disease rather than the study of health. In my opinion, the government should fund research for alternative approaches. The Singapore government has started a nationwide physical activity programme called the National Steps Challenge, where participants are encouraged to walk while the government analyses the data. This is a great example of how governments can broaden their research to include new alternatives.

Working in the wellness model

> If you want to know how you thought about health, look at your body now. If you want to know how you will look in three years, consider how you think about health today.
>
> —Deepak Chopra, *The Seven Spiritual Laws of Success*

Practitioners in the wellness model have a different perspective on the human body than those in the emergency and rehabilitation models. I feel this is important because it changes the therapy and its outcome. The therapists work with the self-healing mechanism, the innate intelligence of the body, taking no credit for "fixing" people, because they acknowledge that the body's intelligence does the work. Wellness therapists help restore your body's intelligence, while medical practitioners destroy disease. Practitioners in the wellness model include nutritionists and dietitians; chiropractors and osteopaths; physical therapists; personal coaches, counselors and meditation teachers; massage therapists, kinesiologists, and foot reflexologists; staff at detox and health centres; teachers of yoga, Pilates, and tai chi; as well as those who are practitioners of traditional Chinese medicine and other alternative approaches.

These therapies are often dismissed with statements like, "That doesn't work," or "I don't believe in that." This is because the issues they work on are often a lot more subtle than the ones found in fully progressed sicknesses. Wellness practitioners only use medical words (diagnosis) as a form of communication so that we all know what we are talking about. The medical world invented names for diseases and claims to cure them. Wellness practitioners make no such claims. However, because of their Western medical training and intense long-term focus on sickness and fixing disease, it can be difficult for regular doctors to understand the wellness model. Traditional medical doctors treat diseases, while wellness practitioners specialise in health. We definitely need both. For example, to claim that you are working in the wellness model by offering a patient an aspirin to thin the blood and protect them from heart disease is simply not what wellness is about—absolutely not. Cardiologists fix your heart attack but don't make you healthy—much as a fireman will save your burning house, but probably won't come around the next day to repair your burnt book shelf.

As I entered this model, the way I lived my life began to change. I know now, twenty-three years after my sickness, that the changes have influenced the quality of my life in a positive way. Here is a list of personal changes that I made that have worked for me. I am not recommending them to you because I do not know your body. The path to wellness is quite personal. Furthermore, people's needs and daily habits often vary. Developing wellness patterns is not set in stone. Changes that I made included the following.

- I set and achieved the long-term goal of running a marathon.
- I started to stretch my body by attending a weekly yoga class.
- I began buying organic food to keep chemicals out of my body.
- I started drinking more filtered water, less coffee, and less alcohol.
- I took whole-food supplements that made sense to me.
- I became a vegetarian.
- I began to meditate regularly.

The "medicine" consumed in this model is not medicine as you know it, but rather various elements that make your body work better naturally.

These may include regular chiropractic adjustments, whole-food multivitamin or multi-mineral supplements, oil supplements from omega 3, 6 and 9 essential fatty acids, antioxidant supplements to counter the buildup of free radicals (the toxins that age the body), organic fruits and vegetables and juices, and meat raised without added hormones.

There is an enormous difference between taking medicine in model one and taking "medicine" in model three. In model one you swallow, inject or inhale a specific type of medicine for a specific disease. For example, an asthma sufferer inhales medication to alleviate the symptoms of an asthma attack; a diabetic injects insulin to help regulate blood sugar levels; a person suffering from high blood pressure swallows diuretics to help keep the blood pressure at safe levels; a person with osteoarthritis may take painkilling medication to make life more bearable; a person with a heart arrhythmia may swallow beta blockers to regulate their heartbeat. These medicines, for the most part, achieve what they claim they do: they address symptoms. A specific medicine is taken to counter a specific symptom. The problem is that the cause is masked.

In the wellness model, the "medicine" is taken so that the body, as an organism, has the best possible chance of functioning well. Vitamins are not taken to treat high blood pressure; essential fatty acids are not taken to make the heart beat better. We don't avoid foods high in sugar to cure diabetes. We don't breathe good air to avoid or treat asthma. It seems logical that maintaining a healthy body weight, having stress management procedures in place and eating good fats may help the heart function. Does it not make sense that controlling blood sugar levels to minimise extreme peaks and valleys will cause less stress to the pancreas and therefore help it function better? Or that by reducing your body weight you may reduce the strain on every joint in your body and therefore help slow down the process of osteoarthritis? In the wellness model, the attitude is not about treatment, it is about self-care and healthcare. Arthritis in the low back is a great example, because sooner or later we all suffer from it. If you keep your spine healthy with exercise, chiropractic care, decent posture and an optimal body weight, it will degenerate far more slowly than the spine of an overweight person who doesn't exercise, sits at a desk staring at a monitor all day long for years, and receives no chiropractic adjustments.

Many people think that the wellness model is too difficult to incorporate into their everyday life. My suggestion is to begin simply and with ease. Start with an extra hour of sleep, or say no to one extra coffee or beer or cigarette. Or try walking to the grocery store the long way. These things are not difficult in themselves but to make them a habit takes time, commitment and consistency. In the beginning, it can be hard to change your pattern from a short-term, crisis-focused destructive model to one of greater human potential. But the reality is that the roller-coaster crisis model is the most difficult on your body in the long run.

Of course, living in the wellness model does not guarantee that you will not get sick. However, adopting this model will increase your chance of being truly healthy. The most common reason for lost health comes down to lifestyle, and your lifestyle is well within your control. Furthermore, statistics show that it is worth embracing the wellness model. Overweight or chronically overstressed people have a greater chance of suffering problems with heart function; chronically dehydrated people suffer more from lethargy than those who drink water regularly; mature adults who don't stretch regularly suffer more from stiffness, aches and pains than those who go to a yoga class regularly; people whose busy lifestyle does not incorporate time for relaxing are often emotionally irritated. These are not judgments on whether they are good or bad people. It is just that, over time, cause leads to effect like a chain reaction. Remember, the wellness model includes nothing that your rational logical mind can honestly argue against. Understood and used properly, the wellness model is a sound approach for the long term.

Beyond the three models: a vitalistic perspective

More than a separate healthcare model, vitalism is a belief system that can run through all healthcare models. If you believe that your body has its own innate intelligence, you have a vitalistic perspective. If you carry this into any of the healthcare models, you will approach any treatment or lifestyle tweaks that you make with the idea of supporting the intelligence of your body. Vitalists seek out ways to assist the natural intelligence of their body. We'll explore vitalism more in chapter 4.

For the moment, though, let's move on and discover the "undoctored" lifestyle. When I filled out the forms for a new health insurance plan last week, I realised I had not consulted a practitioner of Western medicine since 1997. Living the undoctored life is really a possibility.

Chapter 3

Living the Undoctored Life

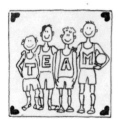 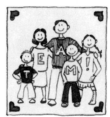 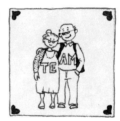

You can't be that kid standing at the top of the water slide
overthinking it. You have to go down the chute.

—Tina Fey, actress, writer, and producer

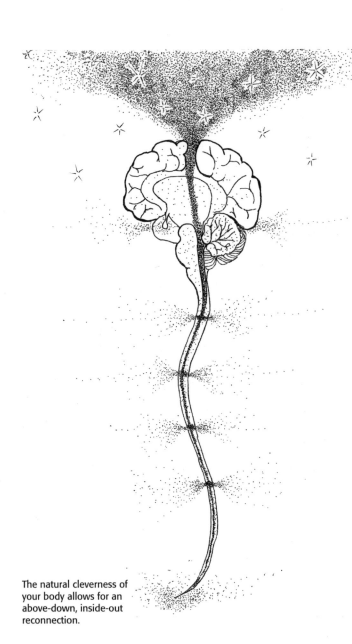

The natural cleverness of
your body allows for an
above-down, inside-out
reconnection.

My dad always said, "You've gotta create the play, son; you've gotta make things happen," while playing Australian football with me when I was a kid. Every Sunday in winter, he would take me to play footy in rain, hail or sunshine. I was too young then to realise how strong my dad's influence was. Profound yet basic childhood lessons and memories often re-emerge in your adult life in a timely fashion. As I get older, I enjoy connecting the dots that make sense of the path I have taken and the decisions that I have made. My father's advice rings true to the wellness model of healthcare and creating your personal wellness team around you: you've got to *do* it, rather than just thinking about doing it.

In 1996, Western medical doctors literally saved my life. Since then, I have not visited a conventional doctor and have essentially lived an undoctored life. Of course, if I have an emergency, I will need a hospital, but fortunately this has not happened to me.

Health comes from the inside, not the outside

The doctor of the future will give no medicine, but will interest his patients in the care of the human frame, in diet, and in the cause and prevention of disease.

—American inventor Thomas Edison (1847–1931)

There are several bases to cover if you want to maximise the possibility of maintaining health and avoiding disease. Remember, disease is only the loss of health. Diseases may result from low immunity or from actions and a lifestyle that do not promote health. Our basic underlying premise is to focus on health, not sickness. I make no claims about curing disease; I focus on raising your health.

Luckily, thanks to consumer demand over the past decades, making positive choices is easier than it ever has been. Consumer demand is a powerful force and it does change market conditions, especially in the health industry. Think of hippies in the late sixties, eating organic vegetables, breastfeeding their children for at least twelve months, doing yoga, wearing handmade clothing, and choosing to turn away from the hectic and stressful life that the average consumer was embracing. They blazed the trail for the booming wellness industry of today. Just look at what has happened in Singapore this past fifteen years: organic food is more readily available; yoga and Pilates studios are popping up all over the place; wellness practitioners are more in demand now than ever before as modern-day consumers seek more holistic care for their bodies and minds. Some health insurance companies offer discounts to consumers embracing a wellness lifestyle by not smoking or not eating meat; consumers are assuming more control of the medications they take; detoxifying juice and supplement kits can be purchased at regular supermarkets; and wellness spas offering all kinds of detox programmes are increasingly prevalent.

Self-care and wellness care

The undoctored life begins with self-care and wellness care. As my dad always said, "you've gotta create the play" by getting used to new habits that will enhance your health. One of the problems for people with poor health habits is that the results of their bad habits don't show up until much later in life. The fact is that if you keep on doing things a certain way, you will always get the same predictable result. Negative habits breed negative consequences; positive habits breed positive consequences. Have you noticed that your habits also create a momentum in a certain direction? Bad habits create more bad habits, while good ones breed other good habits. For example, if you are stressed, you could drink alcohol to help you sleep. This will inevitably lead to overeating, poorly controlled emotions and a lack of motivation for exercise. Start going to the chiropractor, on the other hand, and I bet you will start exercising, make better food choices and drink more water.

Self-care consists of activities that you can easily do yourself. You do not need professional advice to do them. The list I have made here is by no means complete, but it will give you an idea where to begin. Bear in mind that self-care is fundamental to health. It is also the least expensive measure you can take, in both the short and the long term. It's also the most convenient, because you can practice self-care in the context of your daily life. You don't need to set aside hours of your precious time to be healthy.

The other fundamental aspect of health—wellness care—involves building a team of wellness professionals to support you. In English, the word TEAM could stand for Together Everyone Achieves More, and this is certainly how wellness care works. You do not have to be alone in your pursuit of health. It is far easier to consult health practitioners trained in wellness and vitalistic principles. Seek out practitioners who you feel comfortable with, so you will be able to trust them and you will understand their approach. Consistency is a real key—I suggest working with a practitioner for at least twelve months to give their approach time to find its way into your body.

Self-care through posture

Self-care starts with self-awareness. Let's start with the structure of your body. When you sit, try to have your upper-body weight resting evenly on both of your sit bones. This puts your body at greater ease and costs you less energy. To sit this way, you must keep your legs uncrossed. Sitting in a chair with one leg crossed over the other creates a spiral pattern in your spine and invites degeneration of your spine and pelvis. The worst consequence, though is that your spinal cord becomes twisted over time, reducing the flow of every message that travels along the highway of the spine from your brain to your body and back. When you stand, the same concepts apply: stand evenly on both legs.

I'm not saying you need to sit like a Himalayan monk or stand straight like a soldier. Just relax with your posture, but allow your upper body to rest on an even foundation. If you observe people standing in place—say, in the line at the supermarket, for example—you will notice that most of them are leaning on one leg, which invites lower back and hip degeneration. Just like your house, your body needs a reliable and stable foundation.

Self-care through physical activity

In choosing activities that help keep your heart healthy, your mind clear, your spirit alive and your social life active, I find it helpful to consider their lifetime value. Will you still be able to do a given sport at an older age? Chances are that if you can do it both at the age of twenty-five and at age sixty-five, then that sport does not put too much strain on your body.

The right kind of exercise programme applied over time brings many benefits. But misapplied, it can just be like any other stressor. I see young people enjoying high-contact sports, the disastrous consequences of which don't show up in the body for years to come. If exercise is unpleasant, sooner or later you'll stop doing it. Less intense activities will get you fit without the no-pain-no-gain nonsense.

How about walking? It gets you outside, it doesn't damage your joints, and you can still do it at a ripe old age. Sounds a little boring, I know, but give it a try. You can do it alone or with other people. The long walks that I take with Jyoti, my partner, serve as a strong backbone to our relationship and life planning. When you walk, your heart rate increases, so more oxygen gets to your brain and you can think more clearly. Walking aids digestion, increases blood flow and indirectly helps move toxins out of your body.

To encourage you to walk, one gadget that has become very popular is the step counter, an app that comes ready installed on most smartphones. Try and take at least 10,000 steps a day: this will get you moving away from the sedentary lifestyle that leads to premature aging. Another option to consider is getting a dog, especially if you don't live in the city. A dog needs to be walked several times a day and can act as a motivator for walking no matter whether it's rainy or sunny.

Another option is to join a gym or get a personal trainer. These days, gyms offer great value for your money. Most of them offer in-house specialists who can advise you on a wide range of activities. State-of-the-art equipment makes it easy for you to stay safely within your body's limits, thus preventing injuries. The gym can be a great place to keep your body toned and your physical structure balanced.

You could also try yoga or Pilates. By about the age of twenty-five, your body begins to lose its natural level of flexibility, especially in men. A simple test: try touching your toes. If you cannot reach them, consider giving yoga a try. There are many different styles of yoga; one of them is bound to appeal to you. The best way of becoming acquainted with yoga is to do a test class. Search the Internet for some information or pick up one of the many yoga magazines that are out there. It may take a while for you to find your way in the world of yoga, with all its different levels, techniques, teaching styles, philosophies and instructors. But I'm here to tell you that yoga works. Yoga allows the spirit of life (i.e., your body's innate intelligence) to flow through you. It stills the mind, connects you with your body, increases your flexibility, improves your posture, enhances your breathing and can help with good sleep. Yoga also helps with the release of endorphins and therefore gives you a satisfied feeling. It's great for kids, offering a way for them to get acquainted with their body, and you can keep on doing it well into old age. Compare two people of any age, one with and one without at least five years of yoga, and you will notice a remarkable difference.

Try doing yoga weekly for at least a year without giving up. Do it consistently to get the best results. If you find an instructor you trust and feel comfortable with, they will become a pillar of your wellness team. An experienced and alert yoga instructor has a deep understanding of the body. I touch bodies all day long as a chiropractor, and I know that the spine of a yoga practitioner feels so much more vital than that of a person who doesn't do yoga. I hope that, in the future, health insurance companies realise the importance of practicing yoga with qualified instructors and encourage it.

Self-care through energy management

Manage your energy so you are sure to have enough when it's needed. You've undoubtedly heard of time management, but you are probably less familiar with energy management. Like time, your energy is an essential resource that does not take care of itself, especially as you age. Your energy is what you bring to your family, friends and work, so you need to make sure it is available when it's required. Think of your energy as consisting of four main parts:

Physical energy—Stay fit and healthy and be vigilant about not wearing your body out. Your physical energy is fed by sports, fresh food, and sufficient deep sleep. This means you can't overeat, get drunk on a regular basis, be texting on your phone in the middle of the night, and so on.

Mental energy—Stay mentally composed (easier said than done) and get acquainted with what fatigues your mind. Are you mentally sharper in the morning or evening? What foods make you want to sleep? Do you need music or silence to stay focused?

Emotional energy—Two main areas to keep in check are your home and your work life. If you've had a stressful time at work, you need to find a way to pull it together before you return home. Your family deserves your first-hand energy, not worn-out secondhand energy. The reverse applies for work. If trouble is brewing at home, you need to make your commute to the office count so that you are able to leave your private problems out of your work.

Spiritual energy—Don't squander your spiritual energy either. Your spirit gives rise to your physical, mental and emotional energy. There is no need to prioritise your spiritual energy too much, but if you totally ignore it, you will wake up when you are seventy and have regrets that you did not acknowledge this part of yourself. I'm not talking about organised religion—just having a connection with something much larger than yourself. As you approach your imminent death, your spiritual energy will naturally heighten. I have had the advantage of almost dying, which gave me a perspective that made me look at my life differently. Neglecting your spiritual energy means living your life through your mind, which makes for a miserable existence. The average human has an astonishing 100,000 thoughts a day, and most of them are pure craziness.

Self care through a lifestyle assessment

Luckily for all of us, technology is entering the wellness industry. We can now measure and interpret personal data, such as heart rate variability, with a precision that only medical professionals had access to just a few short years ago. You can now measure your personal data in real time, too, so there's no need to wait for an appointment with a doctor. You do however need to make sure you carry out this measuring with the most accurate devices available.

I underwent the Firstbeat assessment, which is based on analysis of heart rate variability (firstbeat.com), but there are other such assessments out there. The key point is that instead of getting a test done to diagnose a disease, you are getting a test done to assess and measure your health. The results of the assessment will help you to manage stress, exercise appropriately and give you personal feedback on activities that help you recover from a busy day. The goal is to find a balance between work and leisure and between activity and rest, and to identify your strengths and areas for development. Of course, stress cannot be eliminated completely, but it can be managed to ensure you can recover from it sufficiently and find a sustainable rhythm to life.

A good assessment will provide you with valuable personal data, including your body's stress levels, the health effects of your physical activity and your personal fitness development; length of sleep; the number of steps you make per day; the number of calories expended during twenty-four hours; and your heart rate variability, including resting heart rate and maximum heart rate. Your overall status is rated on a scale of 0 to 100, based on the data. If you're into that sort of thing, the test will also show you how you stand in comparison to your peers.

One requirement is that you keep a detailed journal for three days. You have to track everything: when you have coffee, work, eat meals and snacks, spend time helping others, nap, have sex, play with your dog, interact with your children, meditate, and so on. The advantage of this is that you can measure your body's response to these situations with total accuracy, and the results don't lie. Your body is intelligent, so it acts instinctively; the assessment results will clearly show how your body responds to situations throughout your day.

I find that the objective measurement combined with my intuition is a useful feedback loop worth acting on. For example, my longstanding habits include taking an afternoon nap and getting chiropractic adjustments. The objective data from the assessment confirmed that these habits are good for me.

A good assessment will also include a pre- and post-assessment questionnaire that will bring some accountability into the report and help you make some necessary lifestyle tweaks. One small recommendation that I got was to go to bed 30 minutes earlier; since my body had been objectively measured by the device, I was more likely to follow this advice rather than my own impulses. We all know we need to sleep more, have less stress, and exercise regularly, but often this sound advice falls on deaf ears because it is generalised and commonly known. Undergoing a lifestyle assessment shifts the context of this advice to you as an individual, which is far more likely to motivate you.

Self-care through engaging with the natural world

Spending time in nature can have a very calming influence on your stress levels, especially in our information-based, electrically charged modern way of life. I have young clients who are as addicted to computer games and social media as a junkie is to heroin. They may, in the future, suffer from a "sign of the times syndrome"—stress and loss of health due to insufficient engagement with the natural world.

Take time to walk along a beach or swim in the sea. Go outside in the pouring rain and feel the water on your skin; embrace a tree; watch the wind blowing on the beach; stare at a full moon for longer than five minutes. Just get out there and feel the elements. Get out of the artificial environment of the air conditioner.

Self-care through mental attitude

Developing a positive mental attitude is another way to enhance your health. No one is positive all the time, but try to steer your general tendency toward a "glass half-full" mindset. The mind-body connection is no longer seen as a fringe idea. Even the most conservative medical professionals acknowledge that the way you think has a measurable impact on your body.

If you are struggling to create a positive mental attitude, try approaching your mind through your body. What do I mean here? Well, the mind has a big impact on the body, and the reverse is also true: the body has a big impact on the state of your mind. If you exercise your body consistently, you will notice a change in your mental state. Your body will use its inherent cleverness to help your mind become positive. Every time you move a joint in your body, it produces happy hormones. Your spine has the most joints in it, so move your spine and you will move your mind. Staying inactive, on the other hand, just feeds negative thoughts and patterns.

Self-care through spirituality

Create a relationship with something bigger than yourself. A big point of this book is to get you to appreciate, trust and cherish your own body's intelligence. To do this, you need to trust "something" bigger that you: your creator. Some call it God, others identify it as existence or universal intelligence. However you name it, find a way to stay connected to your source. It's obviously beyond the scope of this book to discuss organised religions, so I'm not talking about any particular god—I'm talking about the magic that life has to offer.

Sometimes it happens that you become "one," in some rare moment. Watch the ocean, the tremendous wildness of it—and suddenly you forget your split, your schizophrenia; you relax. You fall together. Or, listening to beautiful music, you can immerse yourself in peaceful creativity. Whenever these moments arise, peace, happiness, and bliss surround you, arise in you, and you feel fulfilled. You can make these moments part of your everyday life. Let the ordinary become extraordinary. When cleaning the floor, cooking food, washing the clothes, you can be perfectly at ease, because you are putting your entire self into these actions, enjoying them, delighting in them.

Self-care through rest

Rest. If you are anything like me, life is busy. Singaporeans take being busy to a whole new level. Life is full. There are all sorts of commitments involving work, family, friends, sporting life, never-ending odd jobs around the home, and hobbies. There are also unanticipated emergencies to deal with in life. Your body cannot perform at its highest level for long periods of time: it needs to rest and regenerate in order to maintain a sense of freshness. This society seems to go, go, go, but don't let it overwhelm you.

Although our smartphones are often blamed for our inability to unwind, they also allow access to some great rest-inducing apps (my favourite is called Calm) that can help you relax at the end of a busy day. I often use my app on the bus on my way home from work.

The wellness care team: the bodyworker

Wellness care just means gathering a team of experts to help you maintain your health. They work with you on a partnership level to improve all aspects of your well-being.

One integral member of that team should be a bodyworker. Whether it be a practitioner of massage, acupuncture, reflexology, traditional Chinese medicine or another kind of physical therapy, this expert will help you reconnect with your body. Such therapies can also greatly improve the body's structure and function. You will find that they can reduce pain naturally, soothe injured muscles, stimulate blood and lymphatic circulation, promote relaxation, assist in removing toxins from the body, and improve vitality and sleep quality. Whether they practice a traditional discipline or a modern therapy, bodyworkers consistently achieve amazing results with their helpful and safe forms of healing.

The wellness care team: the nutritionist

The physician is Nature's assistant.

—Galen, early physiologist (129–200 AD)

The aphorism that you are what you eat is literally true. Whatever you ate for breakfast this morning is now part of your cellular makeup. Consider the miracle of this process: you put the food in your mouth, and then your body slowly and silently incorporates your food. The can of soda you drank yesterday is a part of you today, and so are the fresh vegetables you ate.

There are countless books written on eating correctly, but I am doubtful as to their real value, because your diet is very personal. Furthermore, your dietary requirements often change. It would really be impossible to put all necessary information in one book. A knowledgeable dietician or nutritionist can help you make an eating plan that fits specifically with your body's requirements and brings you better health. My advice is to find a nutritionist who works in the wellness model, not one who focuses on treating disorders. He or she will generally track what you are eating for at least one month before recommending changes, considering your current lifestyle and blending your personal nutritional requirements into a plan.

What I look for in a nutritionist is someone walking the food journey with me, not pointing the finger at everything I put in my mouth, but helping me to give what I eat a place in a long-term picture. I prefer a nutritionist who works with whole foods, with natural supplements. Taking supplements made in a laboratory does not feel right for my body, no matter what the claims are. I also like dieticians who lead by example, who make food and healthy living a personal interest and

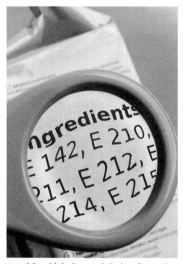

Read food labels to minimise the toxins you ingest.

part of their own life. When you seek out a nutritionist, ask for recommendations from people who have been seeing the same one for more than two years.

Good nutritionists can also help you formulate a long-term detoxification programme. They can examine the content of your stools to make sure that your probiotic, parasite and bacteria levels are normal. They can also do hair analysis to check your mineral levels. I am not a fanatic; I am not talking about Michael Jackson style gloves, or face masks. I do know, however, that we live in a toxic world.

There are two ways of addressing toxins: first, minimise the incoming toxins; second, remove the ones that are already in your body. Toxins can be physical, chemical or mental/emotional. Chemical toxins include alcohol, prescription or non-prescription medicine and food additives. There have never been so many herbicides, insecticides and poisonous chemical pesticides on your food than now. The air we breathe is full of cancer-causing chemicals. Physical toxins come in the form of sporting injuries or injuries from accidents, or from being chronically overweight, for example. Mental toxins come from family-related issues, financial difficulties or work-related problems.

Electrochemical stress comes from computers, radio towers, mobile phones and wireless remote-controls devices. These gadgets change your cellular vibration in the long term. Dr. Charlie Tia, a preeminent Australian neurosurgeon, has spent years studying the exponential increase in brain tumours among children. According to research carried out by Singapore's KK Women's and Children's Hospital, leukemia is still the number one cancer in Singaporean children, with brain tumours at number two, accounting for 20 percent of child cancers. Dr. Tia thinks excessive exposure to electromagnetic fields (EMF) and electromagnetic radiation (EMR) from mobile phones and other electronic equipment is to blame. Scientists also theorise that the radiation given off by mobile phones and other high-tech gadgets may be contributing to one of the most bizarre mysteries ever to happen in the natural world: the abrupt disappearance of bees that pollinate crops, causing harvests to fail.

Every single year that goes by, the quantity of toxins that enters and remains in your body increases. This is unavoidable. The quantity of toxins within a given 10-kilometre area is also growing. In the past fifteen years, electromagnetic radiation has increased exponentially. The number of drugs you ingest goes up, as do the number of heavily addictive chemicals that are added to ready-made foods.

If you are older than twenty, there is a significant likelihood that your body is full of toxins. You must get rid of them to prevent disease. There is no way around it. In fact, if you are currently sick, it is most likely that toxins have made your once-healthy body less able keep disease from developing. Toxins cannot be avoided in today's way of living, but they definitely can be limited and removed regularly from your body.

Avoid anything with the label "diet" or "zero sugar." Most diet drinks that advertise low sugar content contain aspartame, an additive that has been linked with brain tumours, bulimia and obesity. Research also shows that 45 minutes after consuming these drinks you become hungry.

Eat organic food when possible, and focus on seasonal foods. This an enormous factor that will absolutely change your health over time. Of course, eating organic food will not make you feel good instantaneously. But by eating organically over time you will take in more nutrition and fewer addictive chemicals, and you will be more conscious of your food.

When I suggest organic eating, people often comment on the expense of it. Eating organic is generally more expensive, as organic practices cannot compete financially with modern scientific chemical agriculture. But many basic products that we all use daily are similar in price. Look at organic seasonings, organic cooking oils, and the like to make an affordable change that will have a high impact in the long run. Natural salt, for example, has more minerals than industrially produced table salt.

People may also resist organic food because they do not believe "normal" food is so poor in quality and full of additives. Let me illustrate the truth of this. This week on my way to work, I purchased a "healthy sandwich," neatly wrapped in a plastic box. It looked fresh and full of nutritious ingredients, including tomato, lettuce, cheese, cucumber, margarine and carrot, all between two slices of brown bread. I turned the box over to read the ingredients, and found they included the following:

Mono- and diacetyl tartaric acid esters of mono- and diglycerides of fatty acids. Several studies on laboratory animals have proved that these compounds may impede growth, decrease absorption of essential fatty acids, inflame the liver, reduce testicle size and damage the uterus.

Calcium chloride. A synthetic technical aid for additives and flavor enhancer. Risks are bowel disorders, bowel ulcers, vomiting, diarrhea, weakening, shock and internal bleeding.

Sodium nitrate. A very dangerous chemical preservative that is used to conserve meat products as well as to make saltpeter and artificial fertilisers. Risks include hyperactivity, asthma, insomnia, dizziness, low blood pressure and cancer.

Sorbic acid. Research has shown that this additive can disturb enzymatic systems in the body, causing respiratory problems, and skin and eye irritations.

Potassium sorbate. Chemical preservative that may cause birth defects. Risks include asthma, skin rashes, rhinitis and bowel disorders.

Sodium benzoate. This is an additive made from benzoic acid. Risks include hyperactivity, asthma, eye irritation, skin rashes, bowel disorders, growth disorders, insomnia and behavioral problems. This additive also harms the blood; it has been linked to leukemia in both people and animals and it is said to be carcinogenic.

The bottom line: my sandwich was full of poison. Even though it looked healthy, by eating it I was in fact putting small amounts of highly dangerous chemicals into my body.

I suggest you review the components of the nonprescription and prescription medication you are currently taking. But whatever you do, do not stop your medication "cold turkey," because these chemicals are so powerful that your body cannot work well without them. Check out the adverse side effects from your medicine to see how safe they are for long-term use. Ask your doctor if you can have an update and a review of all the medication that you are currently taking. People's bodies now contain a modern-day chemical cocktail derived from industrial chemicals, pesticides, food additives, heavy metals, anesthetics and the residues of pharmaceutical drugs.

Review the ingredients of the cleaning products you use in your house. Most of the chemicals that are in them are not fit for human consumption, and yet we clean our house with them. Cleaning products are often labeled with warnings and the advice to keep them out of children's reach. But these chemicals find their way into your body through your skin or by inhalation. To replace them, there are many environmentally friendly products available that will clean your house without harming you. One simple measure you could take is to use a natural detergent for washing dishes. At least then, you will not be eating or drinking the chemicals in commercial detergent at your next meal.

Look at your deodorant and other personal-care products. Most deodorant states "for external use only," but it is applied to the armpits and immediately absorbed into the lymph system. I know that scientists and the media say such small doses of chemicals are not dangerous. But consider using natural alternatives, like crystal deodorants and lotions and creams that contain only safe, natural ingredients.

Find a reliable source of health information. Keep in mind the basic premise that the problem is lost health, not acquired sickness. It follows then that you look for health knowledge, not necessarily sickness knowledge. Find sources of information that help you enhance the four major pillars of health: the structure of your body, the chemical and physiological processes, the mind and emotions, and the need for rest. Sure, you can focus on your sickness and find a lot of information about it on the Internet. Choosing the healthy "glass half full" as your focus for knowledge is better for your life. Furthermore, trying to diagnose your symptoms from information on the Internet is dangerous. Your doctor may have studied for ten years to gain specific skills and knowledge, so why second-guess him or her? Make health knowledge your focus. There are hundreds of reliable books and several Internet sites where you can learn to be "scientifically healthy."

The wellness care team: the coach

Consult a coach. Top athletes like Tiger Woods (the world's best golfer) and Kelly Slater (the world's best surfer) all have coaches. A coach can help in many aspects of your life; you do not have to be in a crisis to want to consult one. A coach can help with your personal development, relationship development, financial development, life planning and goal setting. A good coach has been trained in models that can structure problem-solving clearly, and will use well-organised protocols while still skillfully giving a personal touch to your specific issues.

The wellness care team: the chiropractor

Medicine is the study of disease and what causes man to die.

Chiropractic is the study of health and what causes man to live.

—B. J. Palmer[1]

I have saved what I feel is the most crucial part of my book until now, partly because this is not a book about chiropractic, but about wellness and quality living. That said, there is one health-saving measure that is an ideal umbrella for all the self-care measures listed above: get long-term chiropractic care in your life. It will greatly enhance the benefits you

---

[1] B. J. Palmer (1882–1961) was the developer of the modern chiropractic approach and a pioneer of integral consciousness and integral leadership. He was the president of the first chiropractic school from 1906 to 1961, and in his life became an author, teacher, businessman, traveller—and for many, the carrier of a sacred torch. Many men and women experienced personal development after coming into contact with him, because he had a gift for bringing forth the innate creative substance buried deep in every individual, allowing it to emerge and be experienced in daily life.

derive from exercise, good food choices, your detoxifying programme, drinking sufficient water, and having enough rest.

Research has repeatedly concluded that your nervous system, when interfered with, causes your body to break down. A compromised nervous system robs the body of its potential. When the nervous system is rebalanced, however, the body begins to work better and repair itself. Good rest, for example, will be of little value if your nerves are not working well. Have you ever woken after a long sleep and still felt incredibly tired? A strength-building gym programme will be of limited value if the nerves going to your muscles have no clear path. Furthermore, high-quality organic food will have less benefit if your nerves cannot transfer that food to a valuable fuel source. Lastly, mindfulness exercises will be difficult if every time you sit down your nerves are screaming in pain.

The philosophy of chiropractic

Chiropractic offers a different and strategically directed way to live a healthy lifestyle . . . See the repair and regeneration of your body as a journey rather than a series of events.

—Dr. Mark Postles, CEO of Quest Chiropractic Coaching

Chiropractic is probably one of the most misunderstood health services, despite its 120-year history and its enormous rise in popularity over the past decade. Its philosophy is very simple. The essence of chiropractic is that healing takes place from the inside of the body. A chiropractor takes care of the nervous system, which controls every single function in the body. Unfortunately, most people seek the short-term services of a chiropractor to help relieve symptoms—to "fix" something the way a mechanic would "fix" a mechanical problem. If you can discover the real lasting value of long-term chiropractic care and let your body slowly show its potential to you, however, you will find that the difference is like night and day. As an analogy, you could use your laptop computer as a place to rest your shoes on while you sleep, or you could plug it into the Internet and find information on anything your mind can conceive of. Treating symptoms with chiropractic care is fine, but it keeps you from accessing the deeper, longer-lasting benefits that regular chiropractic care has to offer.

Give chiropractic at least twelve to eighteen months of consistent use before making a judgment. As a chiropractor, I find that it takes at least this long for me to truly get to know a person's body. Sure, I have completed an in-depth study of human anatomy and all of the important "-ologies" (neurology, physiology, pathology, histology, oncology) but in the real world, people are not frozen in time the way they are on a page in a medical textbook: they have good and bad times, ups and downs in their energy; they fall, they get divorced, they get tired from raising children, and they have times in which they struggle financially. No book on scientific pathology will tell you that an ugly and drawn-out divorce process can ignite pathological processes, but the reality is that it can. That is what I mean when I say it takes me some time to get to know my client's body. It's not that I lack the knowledge; it's that if you are over thirty-five, your body has experienced enough to make it a unique, complex system.

Consistent care also gives a more accurate picture of your health in that your body's tendencies are tracked over a longer time period. Blood tests or X-rays are simply snapshots in time. How often have you been "sick" for a long time when the results of your blood tests were normal? A planned series of chiropractic adjustments with the use of functional progress reports over an initial twelve-month period gives a more in-depth view of how your body works; it shows how your body is actually functioning, not just how it is feeling. And there can be an enormous difference between how you feel and how you function. As a chiropractor, I trust the language of your body (how you function) a lot more that what you tell me (how you are feeling). It's not that I don't believe you, it's just that the language of your body is more reliable. I do notice that the best results come to people who use chiropractic as a part of their life independently of how they are feeling.

Chiropractic is based upon the simple principle that the body naturally wants to be healthy, that the body has its own intelligence which works primarily through the nervous system. When the supporting structures of the human skeleton become misaligned, the nervous system works less effectively in that your brain loses its ease of connection with your body; this could be called "*dis*-ease."

When you use chiropractic to keep your nervous system functioning well, you allow your body to rebalance itself through its own innate intelligence and you will be surprised by the long-term benefits. A vitalistic chiropractor deserves a place on your wellness-care team.

I often hear the question: "If the body is as intelligent and self-healing as you say, why choose long-term chiropractic care? Isn't that a paradox?" The truth is that your body does a magnificent effort at adapting to its environment. Most of the corrections and adaptations are done so smoothly by your body itself that you don't even notice them. But sometimes the physical, mental or chemical stresses people have to endure are greater than the body's resistive capacity. Keep it simple, though: your body either has a tendency toward balance or away from it.

As you become older, the stresses of life tend to accumulate and hang around in your body. I see the body as a translation of the sum of how you think, what you eat, the accidents you have and the dominant posture you use throughout your life (which, for most people, is prolonged sitting). If the external stressors coming into the body are greater than the body's internal resistance, this results in *dis*-ease, which means the body is no longer at ease.

Chiropractic cannot change the story of the stress that caused your body to be in its current state. However, it can change the impact that stress has on your body. Get chiropractic care when you don't really need to, and it will help your body deal with the next wave of stress. Chiropractic work is easier when a person is not stressed or in acute pain. It sounds counter-intuitive to visit your chiropractor when you don't need to, but here's the secret: during these periods, it is much easier to exert a positive influence on your body.

Dwell on this for a moment. Consider the idea that the reason for all your suffering is because you lost your connection with your source— what we in chiropractic call "universal intelligence." I mean *all* your suffering, which includes the pain you experience, the toxic people you let into your life, the personal struggles you experience and the excess body weight you cannot lose. Universal intelligence is perfect. It is responsible for beautiful sunsets, trees growing, birds flying south for the winter, the organised chaos of an ant's nest, and helping you recover from illness. This intelligence is your life force. It's the same powerful, intelligent force that made you when your mother's egg received your father's sperm cell. Everything about you is better when this force is flowing freely within you.

A major principle of chiropractic is that "a Universal Intelligence is in all matter and continually gives to it all its properties of action, thus maintaining it in existence." It follows, then, that the job of the chiropractor is to reconnect you with this universal intelligence. In chiropractic we call this "above-down, inside-out reconnection," which means that universal intelligence enters into the human body via the brain (above), flows down your spinal cord, and powers you from the depths of your insides until it is finally expressed outwardly.

The difference between this perfect source that enters your body and the expression you have of yourself, which is less perfect, is just some interference in your nervous system, which chiropractors as "subluxation." Subluxations may present as tight muscles, local swelling, pain, redness and warmth, or a localised sense of stiffness in your spine. Do a self-test for a subluxation now. Turn your head to the right and then to the left. If you can turn farther one way than to the other, you might have a subluxation. Or, stand in front of a mirror and observe your shoulders: if one is higher than the other, you may have a subluxation.

The conditions that we see within a chiropractic office vary enormously. People of all shapes and sizes, of all ages from newborns to geriatrics, turn to a chiropractor for their ailments. Again, don't assume that chiropractors are working to "treat" these symptoms, however. Although people come to us complaining of symptoms, and indeed often report improvements in their specific condition, the focus of the chiropractor is the nervous system, not the symptom. When your body is out of balance, symptoms tend to appear; when your body is in balance, they tend to disappear.

As a chiropractor I have, in essence, only one objective: to help balance the body. That's why I tend to check your body from head to toe, front and back, left and right. I do this to assess the tension and symmetry in your body. Maybe it seems odd to assess your neck when you come to me for your lower back pain, but you have to bear in mind that there is a far bigger picture going on here than just your back pain. Chiropractors tend to take a holistic view of the body.

Is there a possible link between a balanced nervous system and a better-functioning body? Of course there is! In fact, I view the human body as a sort of "translation station" for all the different stressors we experience in our life. There are several major themes that we humans tend to be confronted with throughout our lives; none of us can avoid all stress. That fall you had while learning to ride your bike as a child, the emotional turmoil you encountered when you went through your divorce—those things are in your body, just as decades of cigarette smoking will be in your body. The tension caused by chronic financial pressure finds its way into your body. That car accident you had twenty years ago is in your body. Your strained family relationships are in your body. Years of sitting behind a computer screen is in your body. All of it can be improved with chiropractic care.

This might all sound a bit too simple, or maybe even like a lofty idea not grounded in reality. But consider these concrete research results from a study of people undergoing long-term chiropractic care. The study, by R. L. Sarnat, J. Winterstein, and J. A. Cambron, titled "Clinical utilisation and cost outcomes from an integrative medicine independent physician associate," published in the *Journal of Manipulative & Physiological Therapeutics* in May 2007, found that chiropractic care was associated with less use of medicine and significantly decreased medical costs. The researchers tracked people who used chiropractors as their first-contact providers over a seven-year period. Based on a evaluation of more than 70,000 people per month, the study concluded that these people had 60.2 percent fewer hospital admissions, 59 percent fewer days spent in the hospital, 62 percent fewer outpatient surgeries and procedures, and 85 percent lower pharmaceutical costs when compared with conventional medicine. These are some fantastic results.

The chiropractic approach

The shape, position, tension, and tone of your spine determines the shape, position, tension, and tone of your life.

—Donny Epstein, chiropractor;
author of *The Twelve Stages of Healing*

A human being is just that—a being. We human beings are infinitely complex, and because of this fact, our recovery from sickness is a highly convoluted and individualised journey. I rarely witness the improvement of a person's symptoms or function as a straightforward linear process. And there is a certain unpredictable magic in all of us that keeps me totally intrigued by a person's road to recovery.

One the one hand, chiropractic is linear and rational in its approach to balancing the human body. Rebalancing the body would work every time if humans were robots—just like a mechanic can reliably fix a car when given access to the right spare parts. But we all know human beings are not so simple, not so linear and mechanical after all. When people turn to a chiropractor, their expectations often don't match the actual reality of what happens because recovery is a convoluted process.

Chiropractic has such a fundamental approach to the body. Chiropractors simply focus on balance. We don't try and fix each symptom, one at a time—that would be like a dog chasing its own tail around. This is also why we don't ask you, "How are you doing?" on every visit. It's not that we don't care, it's just that how you feel is quite irrelevant as you start chiropractic. We prefer to detect and correct subluxations, not treat symptoms. It seems counter-intuitive at first, but by re-establishing some balance in your body, it will, over time, start to feel better, and more importantly, function better. Most chiropractors perform progress examinations to track your improvement through chiropractic, and this in turn inevitably leads to fewer symptoms.

Achieving and maintaining wellness

If the guidance given in this chapter sounds too overwhelming or idealistic for you, begin where you can. As the Chinese proverb says, "A journey of a thousand miles begins with a single step." A friend of mine who is a pilot once shared that, while flying a plane, 90 percent of the time he is "off course" and constantly needs to correct himself. Make your gradient of change small: begin with little increments and you will find that one area of improvement will lead to the next.

Starting the wellness-model lifestyle maps out your course to lasting health. But, as usually happens when we start learning anything new, we get frustrated, succumb to short-term thinking, feel overwhelmed and get off-track. We all do this over and over again. It's OK! We fall back into old habits and forget where we want to go. Therefore, we need to keep correcting our course, just like a pilot does. Sustaining extreme long-term effort is a bit fanatical anyway. You simply cannot do it all at once. Actually, change is more sustainable if it takes you several years to develop a strong base of positive habits. Your health is valuable, and anything in life that is valuable takes time.

Stephen Covey, author of *The Seven Habits of Highly Effective People*, worded it perfectly: "Begin with the end in mind." Remember, your body naturally wants to be healthy.

Chapter 4

Your Values Matter

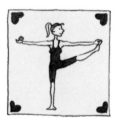

How you do anything is how you do everything.

—Buddhist saying

1. DO YOU BELIEVE YOUR BODY IS CLEVER?
   YES / NO

2. DO YOU BELIEVE YOUR BODY
   IS PART OF NATURE?
   YES / NO

3. DO YOU SEE YOUR BODY AS A HOLISTIC
   SYSTEM WHERE EACH SYSTEM RELIES ON
   AND IS INTERCONNECTED WITH ALL OTHER SYSTEMS?
   YES / NO

4. DO YOU SEE YOUR BODY IN PARTS WHERE EACH
   SYSTEM IS SEPARATE AND HAS NO INFLUENCE
   ON THE OTHER SYSTEMS?
   YES / NO

5. DO YOU HAVE A FRIENDLY RELATIONSHIP
   WITH YOUR BODY?
   YES / NO

Values are the resources deep
within you that help you
decide everything you do.

You bring your personal set of values to everything you do. You might not do it intentionally, but it happens. The same concept can be expressed in different ways, but the underlying message remains the same: "It's not what you do, it's how you do it." A local bank in Singapore expressed it this way: "Every generation expresses itself differently, but the same values define us."

I frequently hear that "opposites attract." This might be useful when building a team of different skill sets, but inevitably it's people's shared values that bond them together and stand the test of time. "Birds of a feather flock together" is often used to describe the coming together of people who have the same interests, but I would argue that value systems are a lot deeper than the common interests you share with your friends. You might be connected with people through your sporting clubs, hobbies or other activities, but it's your deeper values, not your interest groups, that will form your longstanding relationships.

About twenty years ago I met up with an old friend who had a dream of building an eco-village in Byron Bay, on the east coast of Australia. After a decade of working day and night on his environmental utopia, he threw in the towel. I asked him, "If you could start it again, what would you do differently?" His answer has stuck with me, because its truth hit me hard. He said, "I wouldn't establish a community based only on topics that people are interested in [in this case the environment], because something deeper runs people's lives over time. Values surface, and if they are not shared, the project will not stand the test of time. Interest groups may have substance, but over time, it's the affinity to values that helps the group gain lasting traction and momentum."

You and your friends might share similar hobbies like playing golf, flying kites, stamp collecting or cooking. But reflect for a moment that your true friends from your interest groups do in fact share the same values. Interests alone are not enough to keep you together over the long term. Your values are what you stand for and what you believe in. They are the "true north" of your being; they act like an internal compass. Values are the resources deep within you that help you decide everything you do. They form the foundation of the life you live; they shape your destiny. Values are not merely a lofty ideal concept; they cause a knock-on effect in that they produce real results and actions in your life.

Our daily habitual thoughts determine our actions. These actions lead, inevitably, to success or failure, fulfillment or frustration, health or sickness. One of the universal truths in life is that the way you do one thing in your life is the way you do all things. The major areas of your life include family, health, finances, religion, career and hobbies. The level of responsibility you show in raising your children is probably similar in value to the level of responsibility you commit to your health. If you have a crisis in one of the major areas of your life, there is a chance that other areas are in crisis as well. For your long-term health and well-being, it's handy to at least identify these patterns.

The choices we make in every aspect of life are based on our value systems. Being aware of the values that drive your life choices brings a lot of clarity and understanding into your life, especially where your body and health are concerned.

It's not what you do, it's how you do it

As consumers of both health and sick care, we are bombarded with advice about how to keep ourselves and our families healthy—or cure their illness. Spend an evening watching television and you will be invited to try products ranging from headache pills and weight-loss milkshakes to throat-pain-relieving lozenges and anti-dandruff shampoo. Magazines will inform you that organic products are essential, and that eggs from free-range chickens have more love in them than those from caged chickens grown with hormones. Walk into your local pharmacy and you will find entire walls filled with colourful products promising better health and fewer symptoms. If you get pregnant or have children, you'll receive advice from your mother-in-law, your neighbour, your doctor, and myriad other sources. Go to one specialist and their analysis will tell you one thing, but when you get a second opinion it is often different. No wonder consumers are all confused!

When you are clear with your values, making decisions that are right for you becomes a lot easier and more natural. Using your values as a guiding force also takes away the need to be constantly motivated to improve your life. Motivation is a fluctuating resource: sometimes you are motivated and sometimes you are not. Your values are constant, and they tend not to change from one day to the next. They are like an inborn set of tendencies, though they often evolve from the way you were raised and what you have been exposed to.

When this concept is applied to your body, your underlying value systems act as a guiding reference, too. Every decision, including the more subtle ones, are governed by these underlying value systems. Your values might be subconscious at this stage, but I hope that after reading this chapter, you are clearer about what you value. They are so deeply ingrained in you that if you are older than twelve years old, I can't ask you to change them. I don't ask you to think like me either—I just want you to think. Marketing companies spend millions of dollars and use sophisticated tactics to manipulate you into believing in their products, but in spite of their efforts, you are not likely to change the value systems that were developed in you when you were a child.

The ideas in this book are based on certain assumptions:

- The body has innate intelligence
- The body is part of nature
- The body is an interconnected group of systems rather than a disparate collection of independent parts
- A healthy individual has a friendly relationship with his or her body

These beliefs tend to lie on the left side of the spectrum of the values in the chart on page 91. Let's start by defining these values.

Vitalistic: Vitalism is a belief that "vital forces," often equated with the soul, are active in living organisms, and that life cannot be explained solely in terms of material things. Vitalists share the belief that the body is intelligent. They can perceive the wonders of nature, like a storm brewing or a sun setting, in magical ways, fully experiencing the interconnectedness and energy of everything in such moments. Einstein once said, "You can view everything as a miracle or nothing as a miracle." I understand this to mean that you can view life vitalistically or mechanistically.

Mechanistic: At the other end of the spectrum from vitalism, mechanism relates to theories which explain phenomena in purely physical or deterministic terms. For the mechanist, the body has no clever intelligence or soul; everything related to the body can be explained in physical terms. For example, a mechanist will often go to the doctor and get their condition "fixed" by taking chemicals in the form of medicine.

Naturalistic: In the context of this book, I use this term for people who believe their body is a part of nature. A naturalist believes that they are not separate from nature.

Non-naturalistic: At the other end of the spectrum is the belief that humans are separate from nature, and an affinity for items that are made or produced by human beings rather than occurring naturally, especially items that are a copy of something natural.

Holistic: Holism refers to the theory that all of your body parts are in intimate interconnection, such that they cannot exist independently of the whole, or cannot be understood without reference to the whole, which is thus regarded as greater than the sum of its parts.

Reductionistic: In contrast to a person with a holistic view, a reductionist analyses and describes a complex phenomenon in terms of its simple or fundamental constituents. From a body perspective, reductionists seek to understand the whole body by studying the smallest possible part. Germ theory and gene theory are good examples of reductionism.

Humanistic: In this context, a humanist is friendly and has a friendly relationship with their own body.

Authoritarian: At the opposite end of the spectrum from a humanist, an authoritarian shows a lack of concern for the wishes or opinions of others. An authoritarian attitude is very biased toward a person's own methods and points of view.

Examples of beliefs on these four spectrums abound. A holistic person might make their food choices bearing animals or farming methods in mind, whereas a reductionist would not necessarily relate food choices to the way a particular food is produced. A naturalist will enjoy camping and being fully immersed in nature, will enjoy outdoor sports and will wear clothing made from natural fabrics, in natural colours. The non-naturalist will enjoy indoor sports and be drawn to synthetic fabrics and colours. The humanist will be curious about you but will never put you on a pedestal, whereas the authoritarian will praise you or discredit you to their family and friends based on the results you help them produce. The humanist will take responsibility for their life while the authoritarian will blame or thank you for their failures and success. A vitalistic artist will tune into the "zero point field" to help them allow art to "pass through them," while the mechanicistic artist will be concerned about their mechanical technique. Vitalists will have an intimate connection with their soul, whereas mechanists don't believe there is a soul in the human body. A vitalistic surfer will feel the pulse of the wave and be interested in their natural surroundings and the beauty of being in the ocean, but a mechanistic surfer will see the ocean as a wave-producing machine. Humanists value being a member of a champion team; authoritarians value being in a team of champions. The vitalist tends to view subtle symptoms or ailments as friends that they should listen to and that these symptoms are mostly feedback reminders to help them perceive, act or behave in a better manner. A mechanist will view a symptom as a problem to be fixed.

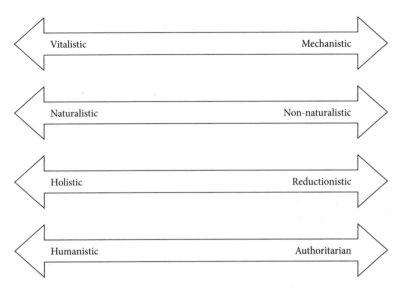

The beliefs on the left and right sides of the spectrum[2] are not mutually exclusive; rather, they encompass tendencies. Although I place myself on the left side of the spectrum, I sometimes use chemicals, take medicine in emergencies (remember, the intensive care unit saved my life) and eat processed food. I wear synthetic clothes sometimes, and use plastic packaging for my grocery shopping when there are no alternatives. But these choices are more like exceptions to the rule. My tendency is to use natural products, to eat whole and fresh food, to enjoy my time in nature and to treat others how I would like to be treated myself.

---

[2] Concept used with permission from Ian Coulter's book *Chiropractic: A Philosophy for Alternative Health Care*, Butterworth-Heinemann, 1999. Coulter is a health consultant and a professor at the UCLA School of Dentistry and at the Los Angeles College of Chiropractic.

How products reveal your values

To get a better sense of where your values lie on these different spectrums, try making a list of the books you love, the kinds of clothes you wear, the doctors you visit, the kinds of food you eat, the sports you play, etc. This will show you a great deal about your belief systems.

Another short exercise can offer lots of information about your values. Go into your bathroom and gather all the products there. I mean, totally empty your bathroom. Put down this book and take 30 minutes to do it now. Put all your products on your kitchen table. Now sort them out by function. In one corner of the table, put all the products you use to clean your bathroom—sponges, toilet cleaner, tile cleaner, window cleaner. In another corner, place all the products you use to clean your body—shampoo, conditioner, soap, bath gel, scrubbing brushes, makeup remover and so on. In another corner, place your personal hygiene products, such as deodorant, face cream, toothpaste, shaving cream, perfume and aftershave. In the last corner, place the products you use to beautify yourself—makeup, eyeliner, mascara, hairspray, skin toner, nail polish, hair removal products and essential oils. Any remaining products that don't fit into these four categories can go in the middle of the table. Put any over-the-counter medications in this pile, too.

Now take a longer look at the products. Are they natural, or are they chemical? Would you use them on a newborn baby? What about the brands you buy—are they brands that use natural ingredients, support the environment, or give back in any way through a corporate social responsibility programme? Are their contents organic? Is the packaging recyclable? Would you dare to eat most of the products you put on your body, or are they "for external use only"? It might sound like I care too much about everything at this stage, but bear with me. Remember the

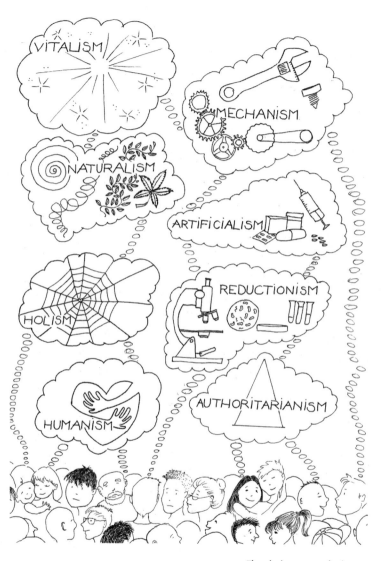

The choices we make in every aspect of life are based on our value systems.

Buddhist quote: "How you do anything is how you do everything."

The goal of this investigation is to see the concrete actions that you are taking at this moment. It may seem irrelevant, but what you have in your private bathroom gives the actual outcomes of your value systems around your health. I used your bathroom because it's not a space we tend to share with the public; it's when we are alone that we are at our most authentic; that is where our values shine through. I chose to start this discussion by investigating your bathroom to determine if what you think you value is actually what you do value. Actions speak a lot louder than words.

For example, you might think initially that you are quite natural in how you treat your body, but discover that all the products you use on your body are completely chemical. This simply means you are not a naturalist and you hold values that are different from what you assumed. As an example, a naturalist's toothpaste would not contain fluoride. If your face cream consists of organic materials, you are probably a naturalist. If you buy from companies because they have a social "giving back" aspect to their business model, you are probably a humanist. Such choices reveal your values clearly.

I hope you find the results of this simple personal investigation enlightening. I certainly do! Most of my long-term clients had bathrooms full of natural products long before they meet me. They don't use natural products because I tell them to; they do it because naturalism is one of their four fundamental values. In that sense, their decision to live a natural life where possible is an inside decision, not an outside one. The products they buy are chosen in accordance with their value system, too, not due to clever marketing programmes that they are exposed to.

Food values

Let's have a look in your fridge. Your fridge is also an honest place that clearly shows your value systems. Do you have lots of fresh food in there? Then you show vitalistic and naturalistic tendencies. If the vegetables you eat are frozen then you are probably a mechanist, because you do not value the properties of fresh food. Do you tend to slowly cook your food or quickly zap it in the microwave? If you tend to buy free-range eggs you display humanistic tendencies, because you show that you care about the welfare of the chickens and their living conditions. Or you might choose free-range eggs because you think they are healthier, which means you show naturalistic tendencies. Are your drinks made from whole foods, or are they mostly artificially flavored fizzy drinks?

I grew up in a stable family environment on the outskirts of a small country town in Australia. Our home was located between the Mars confectionery factory and the McCain's frozen-food factory. (My parents, by the way, are still together and live in the same house where I was born.) One of the happiest events of my parents' life was the invention of the microwave oven. They were such long-term consumers of frozen food that they were invited to be on the testing panel for McCain's frozen meals. They had two huge freezers in the shed filled with frozen food. I vividly remember making new friends during my first year of high school and finding that most of them couldn't stomach the food that I had grown up on, which seemed weird to me at the time. As my circle of influences grew, my food choices changed a lot.

Dealing with the common cold

We all suffer from the common cold once in a while but did you know that the way you manage and respond to it is governed by your value system? I want to illustrate to you just how different your response might be, depending on what values drive your actions regarding your health.

If you are a vitalist and you catch a cold, you will admit that you have been running yourself down with stress or overwork. You trust the cleverness of your body, so you understand that symptoms associated with the common cold—runny nose, headache, lethargy, sweating, aches and pains—are a healthy response to a body that is worn out. You view these symptoms as a clever way for the body to force you to slow down and duly recover. If you are a mechanist who catches a cold, you view your symptoms as a problem: something is wrong and needs to be fixed.

Naturalists among you will let your cold symptoms run their natural course and allow the body to respond at its own rhythm. Non-naturalists will almost certainly reach for painkillers and antibiotics to fix the problem. You will do anything you can to reduce the fever, while naturalists will allow the fever to continue until it wears off.

If you are a holist, you will understand that you are sick because your immune system has been weakened by your busy and stressful lifestyle: holists tend to take a "big picture" view of the situation. Reductionists, however, will blame a particular virus for their cold and will not relate it to the bigger picture of their lifestyle. If you were to ask a reductionist why they are sick they might blame a "virus going around the office," yet will not question why only half of the people in the office are sick but the other half remain healthy. Reductionists believe that germs cause disease while holists believe that the body's weakened immunity allows the virus to take over. Holists will ensure they get rest, that their personal hygiene is in order, and that they take measures to slow life down and manage stress better. Reductionists will focus mostly on fighting the virus with medicine rather than taking better care of themselves.

If you are a humanist you will be quite gentle towards yourself during illness: you will simply surrender to the body's demands for rest. If you are authoritarian, on the other hand, you might get quite angry at yourself and your surroundings while you are sick and those taking care of you might find the job quite challenging!

Please keep in mind that this is just my perspective. I'm not asking you to think the same way I do—I just want to urge you to consider the different approaches to your health, because the way you think determines how you take care of yourself. Furthermore, the way you take care of yourself can allow you to have quite a nice life. Dwell on that for a moment. Doesn't it make sense to you that if you believe that your body is intelligent, if you live in harmony with nature, if you believe your body is a whole interconnected system, and if you develop a friendly attitude to yourself, this will positively influence you in your experience of this gift called life? I believe you will sleep better, be a better spouse, a better parent, concentrate better at your work, and be better able to exercise. I also believe that you will be a happier person. By aligning your values, you will create a life of ease for yourself, because the value systems of the people you spend time with will coincide with yours.

I would like to emphasise that your values run deep, and their implications and outcomes will stay with you for life. There are vitalistic and mechanistic chiropractors, just as there are naturalist and non-naturalist house builders. There are security guards who are humanists, and those who are authoritarian. They both perform the same job, but they are guided by very different inner values.

So please consider that, in all aspects of your life, it's not *what* you do that makes you happy, it's *how* you do it. Identify your values and start living a life of ease by merging with people with shared values.

Chapter 5

Water: Drink It!

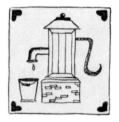

You're not sick, you're thirsty. Don't treat thirst with medication.
—Fereydoon Batmanghelidj, medical doctor,
author of *Your Body's Many Cries for Water*

I hope that you and your children drink enough water and keep doing so forever. We've all heard it before: "Make sure you drink at least eight glasses of water daily." We all know it, but very few of us do it, and almost none of us truly understands the short- and long-term implications of receiving too little water in the body.

To motivate you to drink enough clean water consistently, I will discuss the following in this chapter:

- Some facts about water and your body
- Dehydration: the process of drying up
- The best source of your drinking water: filtered, tap or bottled water
- Twelve golden reasons to drink water
- How much water you need to drink
- The benefits of drinking water

There seems to be a lot of confusion regarding how much to drink, when to drink, and where we should source our drinking water. For example, you might see an article in the newspaper stating that you need to drink water. The very next day you may read exactly the opposite in an article saying that all this "water hype" is rubbish. But the fact is that you must drink water to stay healthy over the long term. There is no real substitute for water.

First, some facts about the clear wet stuff:

- The human body consists of about 70 percent water
- Of this 70 percent, 92 percent is in the blood
- Your brain is 80 percent water
- Your bones are 20 percent water
- Even your teeth are 10 percent water
- You die within three days if you do not take in any fluid
- A staggering 40,000 litres of water cross your cellular membranes every day
- Yes, you need water, and if you do not drink it regularly, you will pay the consequences later in life

For me, water is one of those base necessities that either make or break your health over the long term. Sure, you can find people who swear they are perfectly healthy despite the fact they have drunk little water for more than twenty years. Unfortunately, they do not relate their chronic dehydration to sickness processes. Illnesses of unknown origin, autoimmune diseases and joint-related pains are common complaints for such people once they get beyond the age of fifty.

What is dehydration?

Dehydration is simply the loss of water content. You can observe the dehydration process by placing an orange on your windowsill in the sun. Watch it change as the hours, days and weeks pass by. It becomes harder and lighter in colour, and develops wrinkles. Over time it will smell. Life force leaves the orange. Generally speaking, a comparable process happens in your body when you do not take in fluid. It will not be as immediately visible as it is with an orange, because the orange is a lot smaller. However, the changes will happen eventually. They may be seen locally or generally. Local dehydration refers to one specific area of the body slowly losing its correct functioning; for example, a local loss of water in the large intestine may cause constipation. A general loss of water may be seen as a loss of skin elasticity or dry flaky skin.

The process of continual dehydration is stressful. It causes the brain to take drastic measures and shunt water away from less essential body functions to more important ones. You can function like this for a short time, but not for the long term. It is a kind of slow torture to your body.

Dr. Fereydoon Batmanghelidj[3] states, "I am of the strong opinion that deeply understanding and appreciating chronic dehydration and its implications on human health will create a more affordable and people-friendly healthcare system." Dr. Batmanghelidj asserts that his water-cure plan could reduce national healthcare costs by up to 70 percent.

The average Singaporean office worker needs to alter his or her fluid intake equation. Coffee is a diuretic, which means that it takes water from the body. If we reduced our daily consumption of coffee, we would quickly see positive results. For example, if we were to drop from five to three cups of coffee a day and add six cups of water, this would result in a noticeable drop in the number of sick days taken.

Just try it and see what happens to you. Even if you don't like water

---

[3] Full credit and gratitude for the content of this chapter go to the work of Dr. Batmanghelidj, the world's foremost researcher on the medical properties of water. He was dedicated to spreading the information of new science in medicine and promoting awareness of the hidden wonders of natural, simple, pure water in improving public health and well-being. For more on this groundbreaking pioneer, check out www.watercure.com

or you never feel thirsty, just do it—even if you don't believe me! Do a little experiment for yourself, and just drink more water for the next two months.

Recognizing dehydration

The following is a list of signals your body will give off to indicate chronic or acute dehydration:

Headache, fatigue, concentration problems. Your body's process for filtering toxins becomes sluggish when the body is too dry. The toxins cannot get out of your body, so they continue circulating in your blood and thus cause your body to function poorly. Water is actually the main source of energy for the body. Even all the food you eat has no energetic value until it is hydrolyzed by water and converted to energy. Water is needed to produce melatonin, a hormone essential for sleep regulation. In turn, sleep influences your energy levels.

Dark urine or too little urine. The urine has a higher concentration of toxins when it is dark yellow. By drinking enough water in the morning, try to have your urine a very light yellow by about midday. Your urine will be less concentrated.

A dry mouth. This is a very late signal of dehydration. The strange thing about saliva is that it is always produced upon eating, even if you are dangerously dehydrated. Very few people actually have a dry mouth, so please don't use that as your only signal to drink water.

Constipation. Your stools will harden when they are too dry: water acts as a lubricant to assist in digestion. It is the "oil" in your digestive tube.

A flushed face. The blood supply to the face is connected with the blood supply to the brain. This is an anatomical fact. In times of dehydration, the brain commands a greater share of the available water. The arteries that carry blood to the brain dilate so that more blood can flow through them. At the same time, the face receives more blood due to its anatomical proximity and connections to the brain, and thus becomes red in colour. (This is one of the reasons why a long-term alcoholic has a red face.)

Coffee or alcohol cravings. This is one of the more confusing and tricky ways the body asks for water. You may be tempted to satisfy a feeling of thirst (the body's request for water) with coffee or alcohol. Unfortunately, coffee and alcohol dehydrate the body instead of rehydrating it.

Elevated cholesterol levels. It has been proven that as we get older our thirst mechanism drops off exponentially. As a result, older people drink less fluid. As we drink less, the body develops clever mechanisms to help store and keep hold of the remaining water levels. According to Dr. Batmanghelidj, one of these clever mechanisms is to raise cholesterol levels. Cholesterol forms a sort of plastic membrane around the cell wall, thus preventing the cell from losing water. Isn't that clever? Ironically, we take medicine to decrease cholesterol. (As a side note, cholesterol-lowering medications are among the most unnecessary, overused, expensive and misunderstood drugs on the market.)

If you are suffering from dehydration, you may experience fatigue, poor sexual function, mood swings, headaches and constipation over a short term. Over the long term, you may experience joint pain, sicknesses of unknown origins (autoimmune diseases) and depression. These may all be traced back to a chronic lack of water.

You may not experience any symptoms for a long time. This is because your brain and nervous system do such a clever job of redistributing the water in your body—a sort of drought mechanism. Eventually, however, the consequences of not drinking enough water will catch up with you.

Where should we source our water?

Many people here in Singapore are unsure what to believe and what to ignore. Is the tap water here safe enough to drink? Why does bottled water cost so much more than water from our pipes? Every now and then, a newspaper publishes a research article encouraging us to drink bottled water because it is supposed to be healthier. Then, a week later, an environmental group discourages it because of all the wasted plastic. Sometimes you read about the poor quality of drinking water; not long after that you read about the government's new improved filtration system and ultraviolet-light sterilisation process. What should you make of all this contradictory information?

It is easy to think that you are being healthy by trading tap water for the bottled kind, considering all the benefits that the slogans and the pristine pictures promise: "Free from impurities," "Helps keep you fit and healthy," and so on. Singaporeans are addicted to bottled water costing thousands of times as much as tap water. It's conveniently for sale in every shop that you pass. It's hot outside, so the convenience makes sense, but it comes at a big cost to the wallet and the environment. Most bottled water here is treated in Singapore, bottled in Malaysia, and then transported back to Singapore to be sold. The latest data from market monitors indicate that revenue from sales of bottled water has been rising steadily over the past few years, and came to S$179.4 million in

2018. To put cost into perspective, a 600 ml bottle of water costs between 50 cents and a dollar to buy, but the same amount of tap water only costs 1 cent to make; thus, bottled water is 500 to 1000 times more expensive than tap water. The environmental costs are even higher, according to the Singapore Environmental Council, because most bottled water is sold in single-use bottles. A 2018 study showed that 467 million PET bottles are used in Singapore each year—enough to fill *ninety-four* Olympic sized swimming pools. And the rate of recycling in Singapore comprised only 4 percent of all waste in 2018.

What can you do?

First, check water quality reports. Most local and national water-supply agencies conduct tests and provide such reports to their consumers. Remember that our world is becoming more toxic, and these toxins find their way into our water supply. Determine how good the water from your pipes or well is, and then take steps accordingly.

Second, revitalise your water. (Note: this is for those of you wishing to take your water story further.) You can use one of many water vitalisers on the market, which vary widely in price and specific function, to return your tap water to the same molecular structure found in nature. Energetically speaking, water molecules have a strong memory. Research has shown that water starts carrying the new vibration of everything it touches or feels. It has been known for decades that water is a carrier of information. It is sensitive to medicine, electromagnetic radiation, industrial pollution and sterilisation processes. The molecular structure of the water literally changes away from how nature intended it. It can be difficult for the body to absorb this changed water. The water that comes out of your tap has a different molecular structure than water coming out of a spring. I can attest to this personally, having lived on Tasmania about twenty years ago. This pristine island off the south coast of Australia is famous for its spring water. The energy and life force that I felt when drinking out of those springs was amazing. I could literally feel pure nature in my body, and my body loved this purity.

A beautifully illustrated book called *The Miracle of Water* by Masaru Emoto also demonstrates these differences. This book gives a photographic look at what happens to water's structure when it is not left as nature intended it to be.

Another measure you can take is to flush your pipes. Some buildings in Singapore are old and therefore have either lead or copper pipes to carry drinking water. If you suspect copper contamination (one sign is blue stains around your sink), do not drink the first litre of water after the tap has been unused overnight or for several hours during the day. Let the tap run for a bit to flush the pipes before you fill your glass.

Also, always remember to take water with you when you are out and about. Use a washable glass or steel bottle (water bottles made of regular plastic can harbor high levels of bacteria if left at room temperature over the course of the day, and cannot withstand the heat of a dishwasher).

Finally, you can filter your water. There are pros and cons to this. I figure that your water will get filtered eventually, either by a water filter before it enters your body, or by your liver and kidneys after entering your body. I prefer to filter it beforehand, using a water filter, because the filtration process helps avoid unnecessary chemical pollutants entering the body. There are many types of filter on the market. Their price difference depends on the functions of the filter and the technology used. The simplest form is a refillable water filter jug, which holds about one litre of water. These jugs are portable, which makes them easy to use, and most have a warning system when the filters need replacing. They are an effective way of reducing the heavy metals in your water.

There are also countertop water filters, which you can install next to your sink. These usually have a reverse-osmosis filter system, a PH alkaliser, and a mineral replenisher. I like these devices because they remove chlorine (you can smell this in Singapore's water), lead, pesticides, and herbicides from the water. With these devices, your water is 97 percent free from impurities. It is attached to your normal kitchen plumbing and electricity so it is very convenient. Critics of the reverse-osmosis filter system claim that the natural mineral content of the water is removed but these devices add minerals back into the water before it leaves the filter.

Let me take a moment to talk about bottled water. I believe a healthcare system should support the environment while simultaneously being affordable and supporting your health. Drinking water out of single-use plastic bottles does not meet my criteria; in fact, it fails dismally. In Singapore, the quality of bottled spring water is less strictly controlled than that of tap water. It is a thousand times more expensive than using a water filter. It costs a lot of energy to transport bottled water (water is heavy!). Furthermore, the plastic bottles are bad for the environment—they'll last longer than you and me! They end up being ingested by innocent marine life and will inevitably enter our food chain. Furthermore, the water inside the plastic bottle is contaminated by chemicals in the plastic that leak into the water. Basically, to water or eat food out of plastic is bad for your health and your wallet, and also for this beautiful planet. Getting your water this way is convenient, but the environmental and health consequences are a steep price to pay.

The twelve golden reasons for drinking water

I knew then that W-A-T-E-R meant the wonderful cool something that was flowing over my hand. That living word awakened my soul, gave it light, hope, joy, set it free!

—Helen Keller, deafblind author and public figure

There are literally thousands of reasons why it is essential to have a consistent daily supply of good drinking water. In fact, there are entire books dedicated to this one topic. For the scope of this book however, a list of twelve short and to-the-point reasons will suffice.

1. Water cleans the inside of your body, just as a daily shower cleans the outside of your body. If you do not wash yourself, you will begin to stink within a few days. The "stink" process that happens on the inside often takes years to accumulate. As the years pass, your breath, sweat and other body excretions will all begin to stink if you do not flush yourself with water.

2. Water transports every vitamin and mineral to your cells. Imagine being a carpenter without an arm; it would be difficult to do your job. You need your hands and arms to carry your tools, just as vitamins and minerals need water to carry them to where they need to go.

3. Water regulates your body weight. Often weight problems are not just a question of too many calories coming into the body, but of too few toxins getting out. The toxic equation works in two ways—much like financial health is not only related to your income, but also to your spending patterns.

4. Water controls your body temperature twenty-four hours a day.

The human body operates optimally at a constant temperature of 37.2 degrees. By drinking sufficient water you keep this temperature steady.

5. Water lessens your appetite. Often when you feel hungry you are actually thirsty. The nervous system is not good at differentiating between hunger and thirst. Most people eat when they are actually thirsty.

6. Water lubricates your intestines. It helps push out your stools and therefore remove toxins.

7. Optimal levels of water improve the quality of your blood, resulting in a more efficient collection of oxygen by the cells. This causes more energy, vitality and comfort in the body.

8. Water helps keep your skin clear and slows evidence of aging.

9. Consistent regular water intake decreases the addictive urges of coffee and alcohol.

10. Water is needed to make the neurotransmitters that allow messages to pass to and from your brain for literally every bodily function. Every single function, from blinking to swallowing to growing hair, needs water.

11. Humans don't have a storage system for excess water. Drinking a lot in the morning does not supply enough for the entire day: we simply pee it out. We store fats and protein, and call on our reserves when we need them, but water needs to come consistently from an outside source.

12. The fluid surrounding your brain and spinal cord replenishes itself six times a day. This fluid must come from what you drink, so consider that what you drink will be surrounding your brain soon after consumption. In other words, your brain's function

is greatly influenced by what you drink and this in turn greatly influences the quality of your life.

How much water should we drink, and when?

The timing of your drinking is, in fact, just as important as how much you drink. This is simply because humans effectively store very little water. Given that your water needs fluctuate constantly, it is actually impossible to give standard guidelines for water-drinking volumes. Common sense and feeling your homeostatic mechanism (see page 23) will help you personalise your specific water requirements. Your body's need for water will vary based on personal aspects such as body weight, the season of the year, physical activity, stress levels, menstruation cycle, current level of alcohol intake, smoking, etc.

Let's begin with *when* to drink. Most people don't drink during the nighttime, apart from those who are older or wake often from mental stress. Having been deprived of water for the previous eight hours means that your body is on its way to dehydration when you first wake up in the morning. Do yourself a favour and drink two glasses of water when you brush your teeth. This will make it an automatic part of your morning routine, so you'll be less likely to forget to do it. Getting into this habit will go a long way towards preventing the onset of illness.

For those of you addicted to the morning shot of strong coffee to get your body "woken up": think again. Having coffee as your first drink of the day on a daily basis causes the complications associated with chronic dehydration listed above. In my observation, the people who think they need coffee to start their day often also need alcohol or coffee to finish their day. Alcohol and coffee both remove water from your body. Starting your day with coffee and ending it with alcohol is a very big task for your body's filtration system; your liver and kidneys must work much harder to clean your body. So, to start with, accompany your cup of caffeinated tea or coffee with water. As a general rule, drink two cups of water the same size as the coffee cup you use and you will neutralise the water-dehydrating properties of the caffeine. Your organs will function more efficiently and last longer if you do this.

Drink a glass of water thirty minutes before eating, as well as during meals, to aid digestion. If you still feel hungry after eating, try drinking a glass of water before eating more. Wait a few minutes and then determine whether you are still hungry. You should also drink water before, during, and after physical activity—and I mean water, not the hydrating sport drinks that have become extremely popular with athletes. Some of these drinks contain dangerously high levels of aspartame, an artificial sweetener that enhances taste without adding calories. Aspartame has been linked to neurological disorders and even brain tumours.[4]

Make an effort to keep drinking water throughout the day. Since your brain exchanges the fluid that surrounds it six times daily, you need to distribute your water intake evenly throughout the entire day. Two litres of water at the start of your day and nothing more after that will not do. Water should be consumed at a regular rate throughout the day.

The benefits of drinking water

By drinking water you can delay age-related changes. In 1999, a group of scientists at the Texas Biomedical Research Institute in the USA

---

[4] Ironically, the inventor of one of the best-known sports drinks died of thirst in November 2007. His kidneys failed him. Furthermore, he never wanted aspartame added to his formula, but because of consumer preferences he could not sell his patented idea without adding aspartame to it. Unfortunately, he chose money instead of a clean product.

made a beautiful discovery showing how essential water is to the body. Working with two groups of research subjects, one of people under the age of twenty-five and one of people above fifty-five, they injected all members of both groups with a salt solution that simulated intense, acute dehydration, which can lead to death if not treated. They then sat each group around a table with drinking glasses and jugs of water on it. The under-twenty-five group felt extremely thirsty; they drank several glasses of water in succession to replenish their water levels. The subjects in the other group, who were equally dehydrated, felt little thirst and sat quite passively. Not a single one of them helped themselves to a glass of water.

The researchers conducted brain scans on all the subjects at various intervals after the dehydration was induced. After the salt went into the body, certain areas of the brain became very active only in the group of people under twenty-five. Within three minutes of drinking water, that group had no more measurable activity in this area. After forty-five minutes however, this area became active again. This insinuated that the brain was sending signals for more water. Your brain wants water on an extremely regular basis and if it does not get it, it will take it from other areas of your body. Interestingly, the group of people over fifty-five did not have the same activity in the brain, and felt no thirst.

The researchers came to two main conclusions. First, that the body starts to become dehydrated after about fifty minutes. Secondly, if you are above thirty you cannot rely on thirst as a signal to drink water.

Your body needs water at least once an hour, every waking hour. To determine my own water requirements, I use a formula: for every 35 kilograms of my body weight, I drink a litre of filtered water a day. If I am physically active, I drink a bit more. If I am stressed, I drink a bit more. If I am doing a detoxifying programme or fasting, I drink a lot more. But as a rule, if you weigh 70 kilograms, you need to drink 2 litres a day. If you weigh 65 kilograms, you will need a little less than 2 litres. Keep it simple.

Despite what the media tells you, let me make it perfectly clear that drinking enough clean water is the best health-enhancing change you can make. Now—is it possible to drink too much water? Of course! For one thing, it causes mineral and electrolyte loss. The body needs minerals. If you drink too much water without adding a bit of clean, high-grade salt, you lose too many of these minerals. For example, every time your heart beats you use calcium. If you drink too much water, you will excrete needed calcium with your urine, causing a deficiency. Heart problems may arise. You see, water is only part of the fluid equation. The minerals and electrolytes are just as important as the water itself.

The Texas study described on the opposite page showed that after the age of twenty-five or thirty, the sensation of thirst drops significantly, even when the body is severely dehydrated. Why does this happen? This is one of the very few questions I have regarding the design of the human body.   Other studies have shown that loss of the thirst sensation decreases with age, and this can lead to dehydration in the elderly, with symptoms such as loss of autonomy, loss of cognitive function, and an inability to pass toxins out of the body through the urine. These factors all lead to disease.

The quality of your health and therefore of your life depend on the amount and type of water that you drink. Disease can do some horrible things to people. I think water can help. Is it the total solution? I honestly don't know. But for your body to work well, it needs to be well hydrated. So just do it: drink water every day!

Putting It All Together

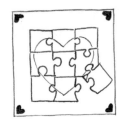

There are no clever tricks or shortcuts for achieving solid levels of sustainable heath. There are, however several simple keys that underlay the process. The biggest key is to focus on health-building principles, not disease-fighting ones. The underlying issue is lost health, not acquired sickness. The solution lies in regaining health, not conquering sickness. A health-based viewpoint—as opposed to a disease perspective—is essential.

I set the tone of the book by highlighting the fact that your body is more intelligent than you could ever imagine or are led to believe. You need to take care of its intelligence.

Then next question I asked was why is there so much disease. We face a paradox: we have one of the most elaborate, organised and expensive healthcare systems of the modern developed world. Yet we have more sick people now than ever. There are more cases of cancer, depression, diabetes, allergies, asthma, sexual dysfunction and hormonal problems now than ever. We need to give urgent attention to our health. It's time to get back to basic common sense and leave the expensive and complicated mindset that has engulfed simple health. I believe that a people-friendly, nature-friendly and affordable healthcare system is the answer.

Your health requirements will inevitably change over time. To best address these changes, it is helpful to view healthcare from the perspective of three distinct models: emergency healthcare, rehabilitation and maintenance, and wellness care.

In addition, there are four major paradigms, or categories of values, that will inform how you approach these three major models: vitalism versus mechanism; naturalism versus non-naturalism; holism versus reductionism; and humanism versus authoritarianism.

The differences between the healthcare models are like night and day. The time factor plays a different role in each model—time is critical in emergencies, but wellness practices can take long periods to show their effects. The costs and benefits associated with each model are very different as well: health is cheaper than disease. The role that modern science plays is acknowledged more by the emergency healthcare model, which focuses on disease than by the wellness care model, in which the focus switches to health. The key is to know which model you are choosing and when to choose it.

Again, I encourage you to relax into these ideas regarding health. Health is not so black-and-white, after all. You are not simply healthy ("normal") or sick. There is an entire health spectrum to be considered. In this book, I divided the journey from birth to death into five phases and discussed the slow change that we make from one phase to the next. Time plays a silent role in the slow degeneration of the body. You aren't suddenly sick. *Dis*-ease—or health—develops in your body over time.

When you get sick, the root problem has little to do with the sickness itself. Sickness simply means that your health has dropped to dangerously low levels—a glass-half-full perspective. Unfortunately, the world is focused on sickness. This perspective needs to change to a focus on health if we want to positively alter the current predicted disease statistics. Health focus is solution-based. Disease focus is problem-based.

Your health rests on four interconnected pillars: the structure of your body; its chemical and physiological functions; your mind, emotions, and spirit; and rest and regeneration. By continually supporting each of these pillars, you will increase your health over the long term.

I established the need for action, for developing healthy tendencies: maintaining a balanced physical body; eating simply and naturally, avoiding chemically treated food; dealing with mental stress; and actively pursuing relaxation. And you don't have to do it alone: I included a number of options for building a wellness team.

I urged you to employ simple common sense when it comes to your health. Although science offers a lot when it comes to disease treatment, I also admit it has limitations. Don't rely only on science. We can "scientifically" prove or disprove almost everything: that we need more or less sleep, that we need to drink water or not, that multivitamins are good or not. But don't you agree that better quality sleep, appropriate quantities of clean water and consistent nutrition make sense despite what "science" proves? Pharmaceutical companies spend a fortune on manipulating results to fulfill their financial goals. I have purposely avoided scientific proof, because science is currently leading us into a more expensive, less effective healthcare system. These days, we have remarkably futuristic high-tech diagnostic machines available to us, but I don't see people getting healthier. Science can help identify disease, but has met with limited success in finding permanent cures.

Finally, I gave an entire chapter to the importance of drinking water regularly. To give yourself the best chance of avoiding disease processes and to sustain your health, you must drink water. You *are* water!

To conclude, I urge you to take your health seriously before it is too late. Disease does horrible things to people. I have been to the depths of lost health; I went to hell and back with my body. I have also worked with thousands of people who would trade all the gold in the world to be healthier. We all deserve to live a healthy life—from the day the egg and sperm that create our embryo meet until the moment we take our last breath. This will not happen without conscious effort, however. Become accountable for your health and family's health. Strive to understand more about yourself and how you, as a human organism, function best. The health choices that you make will affect your quality of life today as well as in the future. In his book *The Greatest Secret of All*, Marc Allen concludes this definitively when he writes:

> Our daily habits and thoughts determine our actions. And these actions lead to success or failure, fulfillment or frustration, health or sickness.

I want us all to live in a world where love and health thrive; where we see our children growing with healthy tendencies and the intrinsic ability to love. I want to see them inspired by the example of older people in society, so that lasting solid health is automatically handed down from one generation to the next.

Thank you for reading my book. I'll continue to do my best to provide accurate, up-to-date, unbiased information to enhance your health. I trust that my concepts have influenced the way that you decide to make your body a better place to be.

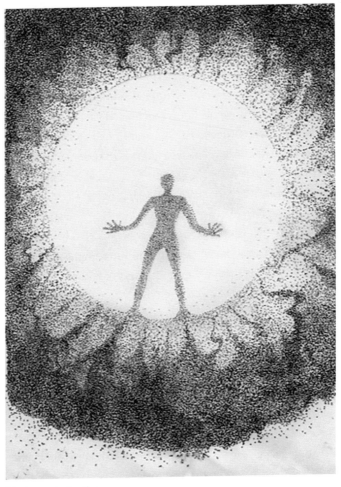

My view, entering the
tunnel of light during my
near-death experience.

Appendix

My near-death experience

In an instant everything went pitch black and I found myself in a vacuum with no sense of where I was. There was a brief moment where I could still sense that I was in my body but that was short lived. The blackness that I found myself in was blacker than the darkest night I had ever experienced. There was no life form either; no plants, no air and no sense of up or down. The silence in this space was deafening. In a vacuum you cannot stand up and the feeling of the normal gravitational pull had totally left me.

A strong panic attack ensued. Where was I? There was no up or down and no relative distance could be felt and I was totally disorientated for longer than was comfortable. I wasn't dizzy or nauseous but I was fully conscious of my displacement. I searched for some familiar objects so I could get a grip of the situation but there was nothing to find. There were absolutely no objects that I could recognise.

Then a pinprick of white light appeared in the distance. Linear distance, as I had known it, could not be estimated in this vacuum and I had no way of knowing whether the light was three metres or three thousand kilometres away. Suddenly, I was magnetically drawn towards this light source. I was not walking or running towards it and there was no sense of gravity at all. It was in that exact moment that I connected the dots of what was happening. I remember thinking "oh yeah, I was sick and now I am dying and I've read about experiences like this." Oddly enough, accepting my death was a very peaceful experience and in that moment I surrendered fully to the end of my short but beautiful life. In an instant the panic attacks stopped and were replaced by total calmness.

As I was moving towards the light source, my whole life story played out before me in fast forward. Every single thing that had ever happened to me was in that film. I saw myself learning how to tie shoelaces as a little boy and how proud I was when I tied my mother's shoelaces for her. I saw the fight I had on the last day of school in grade 10. I saw random smiles from strangers in the street. I saw all the details of the clothes that people around me had worn. The holism of life became clear for me then—nothing that had ever happened to me in my life was "separate" and everything had significance—every single situation, every single moment of my life was supporting me (even the bad bits) and screaming at me to force me to get me to know who I really was. Can you imagine that in one complete instant your entire life makes perfect sense to you; that you understand that your time as a human being is one of the greatest gift that your soul gets? I gave the biggest belly laugh as the cosmic joke of the seriousness of existence was revealed to me. Boy oh boy, this was the most grateful moment of my life.

The film of my life ended without a Hollywood-style finale. My whole experience was flowing and organic with no "parts," making it difficult to explain this holistic story.

I kept moving towards the light source, which was the brightest light that I had ever seen. It was brighter than the focal spot of the sun on a cloudless summer's day. At this point I must still have had some attachment to my body because I covered both of my eyes with my fingertips to protect my eyes. But because I was having such a spectacular experience, I formed small cracks between my fingers to peek through, like a child does when counting in a game of hide and seek. The interesting thing about this light was that although it was extremely bright, it was also soothing. I removed my hands from my eyes and was totally absorbed by it. At this point self love started brewing in me for the first time.

As I approached the light source, its form and contents became clear to me. It was actually the opening to a tunnel of white light and the light had the look and feel of a bottle of clean car oil or the glassiness of a tropical ocean on a windless day. Then something quite significant happened. I could see myself in the entrance of the tunnel of light. This gave rise to the most essential question I had ever asked myself. If that was me in the tunnel, then "who am I, the one seeing me?" I can't account for what happened after that but what I can say was this is when any thought of judging people left me forever and has not returned to this very day. Feelings of unity, the idea that "we are all one," and an ecstatic feeling of self love engulfed me. There were no more judgments of right or wrong, good or bad. There was no more feeling guilty; the whole idea of moralistic behavior seemed so childish. Words like honesty, trustworthy, fair, or well mannered that had concerned me during my life suddenly seemed irrelevant as I realised I couldn't be anything but perfect. We are all perfect.

Before I knew it, I was floating along the tunnel, surrounded by lukewarm, white and perfectly soft liquid light. I was living in the moment and that moment was so full of love that my body barely had the capacity to handle its intensity. My body was undergoing a deep cleansing process and I could sense that I was returning to the source, the very power that had created me. For some inexplicable reason, I could sense a familiarity with the exact moment when my father's sperm cell fertilised my mother's egg to give rise to me. My death linked with the force that created me in a familiar and cosmic way.

One thing to consider as I share this experience with you is that this happened to me 23 years ago. Yet the memory is still vivid, and for me it is more real than the actual life I am leading now. My current life is more like a perfect dream and my near-death experience is the real deal, the eternal nature of my soul.

I continued floating along the tunnel of light. I could never tell you the length of the tunnel because during this moment, no measurements of distance or time were possible. At one point I entered a chamber that had five further tunnels going in different directions. I was undergoing the entire experience passively so I didn't choose which tunnel to continue down and I was drawn to the far left tunnel as though a vortex was sucking me in.

I popped out the other side of the tunnel inside my own self-contained bubble which was about twice the height of my body. I entered into what I might describe as the galaxy. This space was infinitely black, infinitely enormous and was filled with stardust for as far as I could see. There was a vague feeling of other souls journeying with me in that space but we were not together. In that sense this part was an intensely "alone" experience, not lonely, just alone. I could sense the presence of my grandmother, of my childhood dog, and all the souls around me felt familiar, as if I was rejoining my cosmic tribe.

I guess this is the biggest moment of this story. I had touched the light, or heaven, as some prefer to call it. I realised just how lucky I was to have been alive, what a rare opportunity it was, how entertaining life as a human had been. I had so much gratitude for everything that had happened to me during my life. To smell a flower, to listen to music, to be able to study and to do sport all seemed so magical. I could read, go for a walk in nature, make love, watch a movie and go for a surf. Not to forget camping with my parents, fishing with my dad, growing up in the same bedroom as my brother; all of these simple pleasures seemed so magnificent. My consciousness had been confined to a fish bowl and this experience allowed me to feel a million oceans all at once. Life as a human took on a flavor of sacredness.

Just as I was gaining this enormous appreciation for human existence, I landed back in my body fighting for life again. I'm often asked if I chose to come back or if some mystical force sent me back into my body but it wasn't like that for me. The exact moment that I deeply appreciated my life, I was back struggling away in my body. But the struggle was a lot calmer now. After touching the light I knew I had been healed. I knew I would get better and that my exhausted body needed some time to catch up.

Postscript. Three months later I had another near-death experience. I was living in a flat that was above the chiropractic office where I went for daily adjustments. One day, immediately after my chiropractic adjustment, making my way back to the flat, I could sense the same near-death feelings brewing again. Overwhelmed by a bright light, I lay down on the landing. In that moment I knew that the founders of chiropractic were right in their claim that the chiropractic adjustment connects man the physical with man the spiritual. This has deeply affected my own life as a chiropractor. Every adjustment I give, I am aware of its simple power.

Acknowledgments

I arrived in Singapore in 2017 after recently finishing a five-year sabbatical where my partner Jyoti and I had travelled the world while homeschooling our children. Singapore seemed to be the perfect location to continue exploring multicultural living while working again. On any one day here, more than 15 different nationalities enter our office which is the thing I like most about this eclectic, safe and innovative city.

Some special people have made my integration way smoother and I am grateful for their warmth:

My first group of secretaries, Myrna, Rizza and Jessie who have worked in chiropractic for 16 years, with humor, hard work and a love of varied food. Exploring the restaurants of Singapore was certainly a great way to start our relationship. You invited my family into your homes immediately. The care and concern you have for our clients makes my work so much friendlier and easier.

My assistant Arthur. Your professional skills, ability to stay focused and easygoing vibe have been a real anchor for me since starting here. Thank you for always being on time too.

My colleague Sean. After studying chiropractic together in the early nineties, it's great to be sharing the load with you again and to have your gentle energy back in my life. Your understanding of the science, art and philosophy of chiropractic runs deeply.

My illustrator, Heleen Dankbaar, who reached a special milestone. After illustrating my first book in 2009, she suffered a horrific car accident that fractured her skull in many places. Sitting alongside her during her desperate coma I never thought she would survive. Fast forward ten years and she has just completed the artwork for this, my new book. She used the hospital, chiropractic, yoga and the teachings of Joe Dispenza on her road to recovery. And her artwork has so many more layers in it than back then. Sorry for my chaotic direction but in the end it all worked out.

The team at Tuttle Publishing for trusting my message enough to publish the book. I self-published my first book and your team's friendly professionalism has made the process of completing this my second book a much easier process. Thank you to Christina who helped me a lot with the early stages of the book; to my initial editor Alycia for organizing my thoughts; and to Cathy, who helped give more clarity to my expression.

And last but not least, the personal bit—

Our children Dali and Finn; we're on an adventurous journey within the four walls of our family home. Jyoti: my best friend, my lover and the mother of our children. You entered my life at a critical time. The fullness of the life experience we share is magical to me in its own special way.

About the Author

I graduated from RMIT University, Melbourne in 1998. After that we moved to Amsterdam (my wife is Dutch) where we had our chiropractic office for 16 years. My interest lays with family healthcare. I did my post-graduate studies in chiropractic paediatrics focussing on conditions such as poor sleeping and concentration, autism, youth sporting injuries, stress from school, scoliosis, late bed wetting, anxiety and allergies. I also have a key interest in supporting women during their pregnancies. Of course men over 40 and all the issues we face interests me a lot too.

Outside of chiropractic I have several other interests. I've been married to Jyoti since 1999, and we have a daughter Dali and a son Finn. My family loves travelling and we have journeyed around India, Nepal, Indonesia and Sri Lanka, home schooling the children and doing philanthropic work. We are a mad surfing family. We love different cultures and enjoy exploring different foods, music and fashion. I lead a minimalistic lifestyle and prefer experiences over consuming things. Meditation is my addiction and I have been doing this daily for 23 years.

Next time you are in our office, please introduce yourself to me and let me know how I can help you towards a more balanced and comfortable lifestyle. My website is www.thechiropractor.com.sg and you can find me on Twitter @vismaischonfelder